CANCER

SURVIVORSHIP

CANCER
SURVIVORSHIP

How to Navigate the Turbulent Journey

Hussam Haj Hasan

This book should not be a substitute for professional medical advice. The information given in this book serves as a reference volume only. If you use some information, then it's highly recommended that you inform your doctor of your intent before you use such information. We suggest that you always favor your doctor's advice against any literature found in books, journals, magazines, or on the internet.

The information in this book is only meant to guide you through your cancer survivorship phases, starting at your diagnosis meeting with your doctor and into the permanent survivorship phase. The guided strategy outlined in this book should serve as a general path to cancer patients despite the type or the stage of cancer. It isn't meant, however, to answer questions about specific cancer cases. Each medical situation is unique and needs to have addressed particular health requirements and concerns to reach the most hopeful outcomes. Although you may feel that some information here is suitable for your specific situation, we do, however, advise that you run it by your doctor before you take any action.

Cancers in adults and children are markedly different diseases. They are not the same. The type of cancer, how it spreads, and how far it travels in children, is often different than in adults. The information in this book, including advice, recommendations, and guidance for preparing a wellness plan are *not* to be used for children. The child's doctor must monitor the child's progress at all phases of the child's survivorship and offer his or her medical expertise with special care.

© 2020 by Hussam Haj Hasan

All rights reserved. No parts of this publication may be reproduced or transmitted in any form or by any means, electronic or mechanical, including photocopying, recording, or any other information storage and retrieval system without the written permission from the publisher. Please refer to cancerhall.com for more information.

ISBN 978-1-7344921-0-1 paperback
978-1-7344921-1-8 ebook

For questions, comments, and concerns contact

Cancerhall Survivor Network

www.cancerhall.com
www.hussamhasan.com

This book is affectionately dedicated to my mother, who shared in all my happiness and heartaches, achievements, and missteps. Who gave me courage when I felt powerless. Who made me thrive. Your love is my protection, and your devotion is the light for my path. Thank you for pushing me to do.

When I was a boy, I deserved spanking occasionally—well, maybe just a little—but you always disciplined me with your warm hugs and gentle guidance. Way to go, Mom. I love you.

Table of Contents

INTRODUCTION i
PART ONE CANCER BASICS 1
CHAPTER ONE CANCER CONTINUUM 3
CHAPTER TWO CANCER FUNDAMENTALS 15
CHAPTER THREE CLINICAL TRIALS 36
CHAPTER FOUR COMPLEMENTARY AND ALTERNATIVE MEDICINE 46
CHAPTER FIVE SPECIALIZED CANCER CARE 59
PART TWO THE STRATEGY 71
INTRODUCTION TO PART TWO 73
THE ACUTE PHASE LIVING WITH CANCER 83
CHAPTER SIX UNDERSTAND YOUR DIAGNOSIS 85
CHAPTER SEVEN NAVIGATE TREATMENT OPTIONS 98
CHAPTER EIGHT DISCOVER RESOURCES 107
CHAPTER NINE OBSERVE YOUR HEALTH NEEDS 118
THE EXTENDED PHASE LIVING THROUGH CANCER 129
CHAPTER TEN CATEGORIZE YOUR CURRENT HEALTH IN THE EXTENDED PHASE 131
CHAPTER ELEVEN ADAPT TO YOUR NEW HEALTH NEEDS 141
CHAPTER TWELVE NURTURE YOUR BODY, MIND, AND SOUL 155
THE PERMANENT PHASE LIVING BEYOND CANCER 165
CHAPTER THIRTEEN CATEGORIZE YOUR CURRENT HEALTH IN THE PERMANENT PHASE 167
CHAPTER FOURTEEN EVALUATE YOUR LIFE 181
CHAPTER FIFTEEN RESTATE YOUR PRIORITIES 192
CONCLUSION 205
ACKNOWLEDGMENTS 207
BIBLIOGRAPHY 209
RESOURCES 227
ABOUT THE AUTHOR 245
INDEX 247

INTRODUCTION

Your oncologist has just told you that you have cancer. Despite cancer being the most prevalent disease in the world, receiving a diagnosis is still shocking for anyone. You may show signs of anxiety, anger, and depression. Your world comes to a sudden stop, and your life is about to expire. You don't have a future beyond this point. Your mind starts traveling at astronomical speeds, trying to process the diagnosis.

Realizing that you have cancer is harrowing, a nerve-wrecker, and the worst experience imaginable. Your emotional response depends on your support system, coping style, and perception of illness. Okay, enough talking about scary movies.

Your first question after hearing the bad news is, "Why me?" Before you search for an answer, take a deep breath and try to assimilate the information you just received from your oncologist. Although your diagnosis is cancer, your condition might not be as bad as you think. Your diagnosis may render cancer with a high recovery rate—for example, an early-stage skin cancer or even a tumor that could be removed, leaving no traces of the disease.

You are now a cancer survivor. Your diagnosis is the start of your survivorship journey, a new chapter in your life, a period filled with pain and delight, happiness and agony, desire, and apathy. Life won't go as planned, at least not in the immediate future. You'll experience hardship, but if you have the right tools, you'll navigate the turbulent journey with less pain and agony.

This book will help you and your family navigate the turbulent journey through participation in your health and collaboration with your oncologist and members of your health-care team. It will teach you how to draw a case-specific road map for your survivorship. You'll learn the right questions to ask, how to make the best treatment decisions, and how to follow a professionally prepared wellness plan. It will teach you how to make the right decisions about your health needs by using available resources at every phase of your survivorship journey. This book will give you the tools necessary to reach your goals and attain the best outcomes for your cancer situation.

The literature in this book is comprised of research data based on observations and interactions (coaching, diagnosis analysis, case-specific education, and survivorship planning) with cancer patients spanning over two decades. These patients came from all walks of life, with ages ranging from eighteen to seventy-five. Many of them are enjoying their lives, reading a bedtime story to their children or grandchildren, or planning their dream trip (I'm still in contact with most of them). Their fantastic success was the driving force behind writing this book.

Based on my professional experience as a health physicist, a cancer researcher, and educator, this book offers information, guidance, recommendations, and advice for dealing with the emotional and psychosocial aspects of your cancer at all phases of your survivorship. My main goal in this book is to show you that, despite the severity of your disease, there are many avenues you can undertake to tackle your situation and get rewarding outcomes.

Is this book any different from the thousands of published treatises on cancer and survivorship? Would you rather read a book written by an oncologist instead of a book written by a cancer researcher or an educator?

This book offers the most recent information resulting from cancer survivorship research, and is strengthened by multidisciplinary approaches comprising psychosocial, scientific, and medical sciences. In other words, it combines solutions from a range of scientific and psychosocial disciplines. It's a publication that adds to the wealth of information on cancer. Cancer is a massive problem affecting the lives of millions with no telling how or when it will back off. The more knowledge we gain through this book and others, the closer we get to understanding its complexity, and hence, the better the future will look for millions.

To answer the second question, oncologists are doctors who specialize in the diagnosis and treatment of cancer. They dedicate their work, research, and time to treating your cancer. Their education and study rise to the advanced medical level, not intended for the layman to understand. Many of them are well-qualified to write on the subject of survivorship, but it's preferable to get survivorship information and planning from a specialist who possesses the expertise in helping cancer patients with their cancer journeys, a professional with the skills to communicate and have the scientific and medical knowledge to guide you through your journey. This answer does not undermine the role of your oncologist.

My passion for learning about cancer started when I was a health physics graduate student. I began researching patients' participation in their health and how it affects the self-management process of their chronic conditions. It was apparent to me that patient's involvement could not be possible without using a multidisciplinary approach to self-management. This process is necessary to include and prepare the patient to take an active role in making his or her health decisions through collaboration with various medical and nonmedical professionals. It's also crucial to establish an effective doctor-patient partnership to wipe out many obstacles to communications and knowledge disparities. We can only accomplish this partnership through public education.

I intend to help you push ahead despite obstacles to enable you to gain enough knowledge to help make the decisions that matter to your health and wellness. One way to make doctors share decision making with you is by taking control of your disease. You can accomplish this task through dedicated learning of self-management strategies. Your partnerships with your doctors are the only way to enhance your prognosis.

Doctors now recognize how and why cancer emerges and the science behind its emergence and disappearance. They understand risk factors and what they can do to a person and how to prevent them. Now we need to put you, the patient, in charge of your disease to enable you to use the information for your benefit.

This publication is made up of two parts. Part one focuses on providing you with the general knowledge needed to build a wellness program. You can use the information in part one as a reference whenever you have basic cancer questions at any point in your progress.

The second part explains the self-management strategy of your cancer situation, beginning from diagnosis and transitioning into the permanent survivorship phase. Each chapter in the second part of the book revolves around a central argument: Your outlook will improve if you execute your survivorship wellness plan under the continued supervision of your health-care team.

The approach shows you how to locate your position on the cancer-care continuum (chapter 1). Your location allows you to mark the starting point, enabling you to navigate the continuum with a direction specific to your cancer case. Knowledge of your position is crucial so as not to waste any time looking for or researching unrelated matters since cancer is a time-sensitive illness.

The approach to survivorship planning in this book is called UNDOCANCER. Each letter denotes a time interval in the survivorship stage (chapters 6–15). Depending on where you are on the continuum, I will guide you on how to proceed from that point forward. For example, chapter 6, "Understand Your Diagnosis," explains that you must research and understand your cancer diagnosis before you advance into navigating your treatment options (which are explored in chapter 7).

How effective is the program? Does it prolong survival? Does it extend your life? Every cancer situation is distinct, but the strategy in this book (UNDOCANCER) will help you in various ways, including the best ways to plan your survivorship and learn how to always seek a better prognosis for your cancer situation. To realize your cancer demands intervention allows you to manage your own life, and who is a more qualified manager than you when your life is at stake? We understand how to put you in control.

Self-managing your disease isn't always straightforward, taking into consideration your state of mind and potential psychological and probable physical impairment while enduring the agony.

But it's possible, and now we know how.

Did you know you can self-manage your cancer on your own even better than your oncologist? Do you realize that self-management of your disease can produce hopeful results and improve your quality of life? Your oncologist and the health-care team are very busy individuals. Their compassion dissipates after overseeing many patients. The nature of their jobs governs their behavior. They can never take care of you like you can.

Are you diagnosed with cancer, preparing for treatment, or in remission? Are you shocked and confused, unsure of how to proceed from this point forward? Are you powerless and alone? Are you aware of what's next? Despite where you are at in your cancer campaign, *Cancer Survivorship: How to Navigate the Turbulent Journey* is your step-by-step guiding strategy to help you improve your prognosis to provide you with an excellent quality of life.

Compared to other diseases, cancer has defied attempts to find a reliable cure. Scientists and engineers have yet to invent devices capable of detecting the last cancer cell that may have remained in your body after harsh cancer treatment. No legitimate doctor has ever informed the patient that he or she is cancer-free, nor uttered the word *cured* after completing therapy.

Does this mean you must surrender to cancer? The words above should serve as a call to action, toward building a wellness foundation around a whole truth, and should be a challenge to enable you to use creative techniques to self-manage.

There are three different ways to advance after your diagnosis,

- o Commission your doctors to have full control of your illness and try to treat it. Although your oncologist and members of your health-care team will treat your condition as unique, they tackle various obstacles and interruptions while handling other cases.
- o Yield to the disease. If you concede to cancer and think it's the disease that will kill you, you may have a miserable cancer journey, ending with unwanted consequences such as premature death.
- o Or take charge. If you become the manager of your illness, you've made the most rational decision. It involves a hard struggle and collaboration with your primary health-care team. I'm sure you don't mind the responsibility when it's your life you must navigate.

HOW TO USE THIS BOOK

You don't have to read this book cover to cover, nor in sequence. If you have basic cancer knowledge, you can skip part one. Go to the chapter that describes your cancer situation at that moment. However, skim through part one since advances in medicine and technology are progressing at high speeds, and you may wish to keep up with the newest medical information and research. You'll find some repeated text in various sections of the book. The repetition isn't accidental. I've done it on purpose to satisfy the vital requirements of certain cancer situations that might be necessary at different phases of the continuum.

If you're a patient, I recommend that you read all the chapters in part one, despite the type and extent of your cancer and before you dig any further. Besides offering necessary information about cancer, part one outlines popular treatment options to accompany your initial treatment, including complementary therapies and clinical trials. Both are essential treatments that may improve your prognosis and provide you with a good quality of life.

In this book, I will refer to resources should you wish to gain more detailed knowledge about a subject of interest. They'll resemble the format RX. The R refers to the word *resource*, and the X denotes its number. They will appear as superscripts at the ends of paragraphs or sections. The resources section starts on page 227.

Good luck with your journey.

PART ONE
CANCER BASICS

CHAPTER ONE

CANCER CONTINUUM

Life is about a journey that leads to a destination. If you lack the goals to move forward, then life isn't a journey where all expectations vanish. On a business trip, writing a book, during a marriage, and through illness, we make choices to get the best hopeful outcomes from such journeys. They all share a common denominator that aims at goal attainment. To succeed, you must gain skills, inner strength, and determination only possible through seeking specific types of knowledge. Think about the above words; do you see why we categorize cancer as a journey? It's a journey, however unpleasant, filled with elements of difficulty, obstacles, pain, hope, and happiness. Those elements don't necessarily make cancer a fight or a battle. Some of my patients tell me war terminology makes them nervous and stressed. They feel singled out and poorly labeled because of the use of unpopular vocabulary not used in everyday conversations. Other patients felt they are under increased pressure to "fight to win" instead of finding a peaceful way to survive cancer.

Every journey has a starting and ending point and requires planning that could begin hours, days, months or even years before launch. We make plans based on circumstances that could influence events and times within our journeys—journeys related to our jobs, money, and family issues. We plan while wishing the results to be fulfilling and pleasurable. Your cancer journey starts with diagnosis and ends with remission, recovery, or death. Although journeys need preparation before being embarked upon, in cancer, we plan and prepare in the form of prevention and early screening to stop it from starting.

If cancer starts, then your destination, without a doubt, is to seek a cure. So, is it possible that you might become cancer-free? Millions of cancer survivors are living with cancer just fine. They're leading healthy lives. For some, life is even better than what they had before they became cancer survivors. Awareness about lifestyle changes and improved early screening techniques has resulted in an extended five-year survival rate to encompass more patients. Advances in treatment make it possible for patients to experience less severe side effects, leading to less pain and stress through cancer.

A full cancer journey has stages and phases that are further divided into categories. They differ in their characteristics, health needs, and interventions. Together, they produce the care continuum. To move forward, you must meet specific requirements and complete the current stage before you proceed to the next one.

Moving forward is possible through possessing specific educational tools to enable you to manage and pursue extended survival. Knowledge can save your life and help tackle the problematic circumstances before, during, and after treatment. Cancer has a unique position among all journeys because of its ramifications and the many complex components making it a challenging medical phenomenon.

You don't have to experience every part of the cancer continuum; if you had an early-stage tumor that has not spread to adjacent sites in the body, you might get therapy and recover to the point where traces of the disease disappear. The great news is that you don't have to advance to the next level; hence, your journey does not have to engulf the entire spectrum of the continuum in fig 1:1, page 5.

Psychological, psychosocial, and financial issues are prevalent, depending on your health. The accumulated pressure could demand a multidisciplinary team of specialists to intervene and discuss your individual needs and health requirements. Combining the abilities of different professionals from an array of medical, scientific, and psychosocial disciplines can be fundamental to reducing the remarkable burden levied because of the diagnosis. If you think the pressure on you at any point of your journey is interfering with clear thinking, then seek professional help.

The choices you make daily affect your health on the continuum. Many elements serve as obstacles while trying to make progress, ranging from simple to severe. Complications may be in the form of emotional trauma, physical impairments, family and relationship issues, job-related disappointments, and financial matters.

This chapter introduces you to the cancer control continuum and shows what your relative position on it means. It summarizes the stages, phases, and serves as a building block to understanding your cancer. Knowing where you stand on the continuum offers you the details of your cancer situation. Knowing your health situation is vital to show you how to proceed to the next level. This specific knowledge lets you know what to expect as you progress on the continuum. R12, R13, R14

HEALTH ACROSS THE CONTINUUM

The cancer continuum, also known as *the cancer control continuum*, is your cancer lifeline, and it has been used since the mid-1970s to describe the progress of your cancer. You may wish to perceive it as the dynamic, moving part of your journey. It's the gradual progression through many stages that vary in severity. The full continuum is comprised of prevention, early screening, diagnosis, treatment, survivorship, and the end-of-life period. Every stage involves specific health-care requirements (for example, health promotions and medical advice), that could be under influences at multiple levels that can help or impede achievement. Your position, at an instant, defines your present health condition (figure 1:1). The following three sections summarize the stages of the cancer continuum.

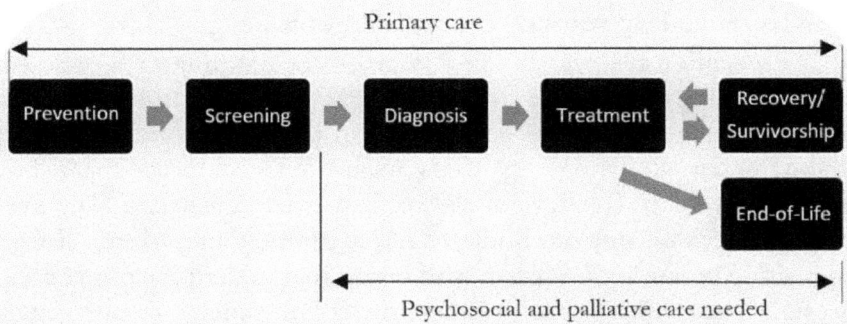

Figure 1:1. Stages of the Cancer-Care Continuum

> The schematic figure above shows your position on the continuum. Primary care is essential for all phases. Besides primary care, the patient may require psychosocial and palliative care to manage their health throughout survivorship. Hospice care is helpful toward the end-of-life period. Find more information about palliative and hospice care in chapter five. R26

Stage One: Prevention

We cannot underestimate the importance of prevention. It helps to stop bad things from happening. It's the action you take to protect yourself against unwanted events, including dreaded diseases such as heart and lung problems and even cancer—yes, cancer. You may ask, "I've been trying to do everything properly. I eat right and exercise, never smoked cigarettes, drink alcohol wisely, and live in a pollution-free area. Why did I get cancer?" Or you may ask, "I've never smoked a cigarette in my entire life, but I have lung cancer. Why?"

Researching the subject can lead to different reports about cancer prevention, where conflicting research data can produce opposing views. While a study provides you with a tip on taking preventive measures, it advises against it in another. Although you may have seen many conflicting reports, the fact remains that developing cancer is affected by your lifestyle habits. By taking a few preventive measures, you can make a difference. Eat right, exercise, don't smoke, drink less alcohol if any, practice safe sex, reduce your exposure to the sun, and have regular checkups. And remember that some risk factors are beyond our control, including age and genetic factors. Cancer prevention is an action to lessen exposure to developing the disease. Through prevention, you also lower your risk of getting a multitude of other ailments, and as a cancer patient, taking preventive measures is also crucial to help you stop cancer from worsening.

Prevention reserves the first stage on the continuum, a period of stable health. Preventive measures against a dreadful cancer are relevant since cancer cells lie dormant in us, and the goal is to keep them that way. Living organisms make defective cells, that's how tumors are born. But several mechanisms that detect and keep such cells in check occupy our bodies. They are not enough to stop it from appearing in our lives. We live with myths that undermine our capacity to fight such disease. For example, many link cancers to our genetic makeup instead of lifestyles. According to research, the contrary is true.

According to the World Health Organization (WHO), cancer is the second leading cause of death worldwide, killing about 9.6 million in 2018. Approximately 70 percent of deaths occur in low and middle-income countries. During the next decade, the number of people in the United States diagnosed with cancer will increase by 31 percent compared to 2012. The World Health Organization also confirms that tobacco use alone is responsible for 22 percent of all cancer deaths. The economic impact of cancer is significant and is increasing. The total annual economic cost of cancer in 2010 was estimated at approximately 1.16 trillion dollars. The only solution for such an increase is to enact programs to control cancer fatalities through education and implementing programs to help diminish risk factors. These programs could pay tremendous dividends on lives saved. Mortality reduction is challenging without eliminating the obstacles of socioeconomic disparities, barriers that limit access to health care, and widespread obesity.

Stage Two: Early Screening

Various medical and cancer authorities, including the National Cancer Institute, the American Cancer Society, and the World Health Organization, refer to early screening as the use of simple tests across a healthy population to identify individuals who have a disease, but do not yet have symptoms. With cancer, early screening gives doctors the chance to diagnose it before it grows large and invades other areas of the body. The detection of early signs allows for improved long-term survival for those with first signs of the tumor, compared to patients whose symptoms appeared after cancer surfaces. Doctors attempt to search for cancerous cells or tissue when no signs are present to enable them to perform diagnosis as fast as possible. An example of recognizing early symptoms would be spotting a new mole and having it examined by a dermatologist to make sure it's not a sign of melanoma, a deadly form of cancer if not detected early.

The problem arises when doctors cannot find many types of malignancies because early detection tests don't exist for many cancers. When doctors find cancer through early detection, they still cannot prove that such an event can reduce mortality. Early detection does not guarantee an improved prognosis, but it can improve the outcomes of specific cases. Patients with early forms of brain tumors, breast, cervical, colorectal, prostate, and skin cancers are most likely to experience improved results because of early detection. But challenges rely on individual behaviors; often, personal responsibility to schedule the mammogram (for screening the breast), pap smear (for screening the cervix), colonoscopy (for screening the colon), or planning a dermatologist appointment.

In those situations, early findings of signs can lead to a better prognosis. For example, when doctors detect cervical cancer early, the success rate for improvement is possible as with colorectal and breast cancers. Although research can be a challenge, the potential rewards—on deaths avoided—make it an essential and valuable research study.

Stage Three: Survivorship

Survivorship occupies the last stage of the continuum and is made up of phases characterizing the beginning and conclusion of the cancer journey. The survivorship period starts when the cancer is detected, at diagnosis, and can last throughout the permanent phase where doctors consider the disease a chronic condition.

Survivorship is comprised of the following three phases; each differs from its predecessor:

> Phase 1: Acute, begins at diagnosis until the end of the treatment period.
> Phase 2: Extended, begins when treatment ends and extends for the following few months.
> Phase 3: Permanent, begins a few months after completing treatment and lasts for the balance of life.

Phases and their categories in this stage encompass the diagnosis, treatment periods, and all the challenges ahead. Each event in this stage is a milestone in your life during the journey for their remarkable impacts. Diagnosis marks the start of the acute phase, and somewhere in the permanent survivorship phase designates the end. Note that end-of-life does not only mean death by cancer; it could occur because of an unrelated event.

During diagnosis, collecting information begins through consultations with your primary doctor and your oncologist. The collection period focuses on learning the staging and progression of the disease. It offers you the chance to make informed decisions on treatment options and other related matters, including clinical trials and complementary therapies (chapters 3 and 4). It is also beneficial to start learning about specialized cancer care such as palliative care (chapter 5). Getting a second, even a third opinion after receiving your diagnosis is vital and sometimes critical. From this point on, you are a survivor, a label popular among cancer patients and medical entities.

This name will accompany you for the rest of your life, even if your doctor declares you as cancer-free.

The treatment period begins a few days after receiving the news of the diagnosis. Now, you'll get one or a mix of the most common cancer treatments, including surgery, chemotherapy, radiotherapy, or one of the less conventional therapies, such as immunotherapy. What you'll receive depends on how progressive your cancer is—for example, how far it's traveled from the primary location, the stage and size of the tumor, your age, and your health status. You may experience enhanced psychological issues because of such a harsh experience at diagnosis time.

Survivorship planning requires managing the long-term and late-term side effects, rehabilitation, and dealing with possible psychological and physical impairments. Your oncologist will help you take the preventive measures against recurrence (cancer reemergence), taking advantage of palliative care and other support systems, and guide you in how to perform health promotions.

When patients transition out of the survivorship into the end-of-life period, they have the chance to decide on palliative and hospice care to enjoy a good quality of life in the remaining few months. During this unfortunate period, this unique support can involve your family members and caregivers. It gives everyone involved peace of mind to prepare for death.

YOUR POSITION ON THE CARE CONTINUUM

You can use the schematic trajectory in (figure 1:1, page 5) to know your position on the cancer continuum. Your place serves as your current health status. For example, if you don't have cancer but are interested in using preventive measures to reduce your risk of getting cancer, your position will be somewhere in the first two stages of the continuum—prevention and early screening. At these two stages, doctors recommend you look for ways to stay healthy and reduce your exposure to risk factors.

Knowing your position on the continuum leads you to the right chapters specific to your cancer. It dictates what resources to activate necessary for your situation. It also reduces your general knowledge inquiry period so you won't waste time gathering irrelevant resources, and it helps you narrow your search to focus only on your specific case.

For example, imagine you grabbed this book when you completed chemotherapy—then ignoring preceding chapters covering the acute period is logical. You'll investigate the extended and permanent stages covered in chapters 10–14. Information in these chapters alone is never enough knowledge for any patient. You must activate other resources through the many available channels and gather as much information as possible on your specific case and health needs. The resources section in this book provides you with specific resources for your condition. Professional guidance is always necessary while searching for answers, and your best source is your primary care team and your oncologist. Start by finding specific information related to your cancer situation; this is your first step toward taking part in your own health decisions.

PARTICIPATION IN YOUR HEALTH

Participation in health should happen at all stages of the continuum for everyone. As a patient, your involvement means engagements in decision making at every phase of survivorship, enabling you to express opinions on treatment options and future changes in lifestyle. It serves as a beginning to the disease self-care. Participation is seen by sharing information with your health-care team. You must have the will to share your emotions, psychological state, and common signs that may help the overall progress. Information sharing during all phases of survivorship is necessary to continue self-managing your disease. Participation demands active duties and responsibilities, along with accepting the task of changing your lifestyle habits into better ones.

Participation does not decrease the role of the oncologist or other members of your health-care team engaged in treating your illness; instead, it emphasizes that to gain success during your journey, you must complement your doctor's role in taking care of your health. We call your engagement *self-management.*

Many doctors have welcomed patients' involvement in their chronic illnesses through partial self-management. Now you can contribute by administering your disease under the careful and adequate supervision of your care team. It's a contribution to reduce the overwhelming burden of the workload experienced by doctors. It also gives the patient confidence in making the right healthy choices.

Patient participation is essential to manage chronic illnesses because of the long duration of the condition. Patients don't self-manage on their own. Health professionals and patients work together to achieve the same goal.

The concept of self-management of your chronic condition is intuitive, and an ongoing daily measure in which you take an active role to control the disease. When self-managing, you may also need help from your family and friends. Everyone works in harmony to oversee and manage symptoms, lifestyle changes, psychosocial, cultural, and spiritual consequences of health conditions. When members work together, they produce optimal management resulting in favorable outcomes. It's an ongoing course of action where everyone involved must contribute his or her part in their perspective fields, providing that everyone incorporates your view.

The National Center for Health Statistics defines a chronic disease as one lasting three months or more. Hence, it persists for a long time. Doctors can contain chronic conditions but not cure them. Cancer can go into various kinds of remission (chapter 13), to where therapy is useful. Doctors can control your situation with treatment, meaning it might seem to disappear or stay the same. A few doctors consider some metastatic stage IV cancers to be chronic illnesses where patients may live with them for a long time. Metastatic breast and prostate cancers are examples of chronic conditions.

Constant monitoring and self-care are necessary to sustain good, positive health to conclude the best outcomes during the self-management process. Doctors always contribute to the patient's case for the duration of the illness, but introducing self-management performed by the alarmed patient allows the doctors to help others in desperate need. The results are great for everyone involved. It's a win-win situation.

You can find more information about the cancer continuum and its stages in the resources section of this book. [R12, R13, R14]

AN OVERVIEW OF SELF-CARE BASICS

This chapter introduced you to a simple definition of stages and phases of your continuum and emphasized their importance in recognizing your position as a sign of your current health. The first two stages, prevention and early screening, are essential for nonpatients and patients alike.

Below are summaries of the essential elements to self-care necessary to help in executing the wellness strategy during the survivorship period of the journey (chapters 2–5). In these chapters, you'll find answers to many important questions and explanations of some confusing details related to cancer. The information in these chapters will touch most of the basics to allow you to make informed decisions specific to your health needs.

Chapter Two: Cancer Fundamentals

As a patient, learning cancer basics is vital to qualify you to become involved in making treatment decisions. Before you make these decisions, you must know your cancer origination, risk factors, signs and symptoms, stages, progression, and prognosis. The goal here is to provide you with the tools necessary for you to discover the next step. After you complete treatment, you must decide on many other issues to help you progress and adjust to the new changes. And to become successful in making new health plans, you must readjust to the new environment after treatment and be able to lessen the side effects of surgery, chemotherapy, and radiation therapy. This chapter won't answer every question you may have, but it gives you the basics to gather resources on your specific case.

Chapter Three: Clinical Trials

Clinical trials are research studies to get vital information on treatments or drugs. Medical professionals, including oncologists, researchers, lab technicians, health administrators, and specialists from other disciplines such as chemists, biologists, and physicists, perform clinical-trial research. Besides the possibility of trying new medical procedures or drugs that are not available to the public yet, they are vital to finding what works and what doesn't. If the Food and Drug Administration (FDA) approves the new resulting drug or development on treatment, doctors can use them to help future patients. They are your chance to try tomorrow's medicine today. Patients should consider clinical trials while deciding on the most suitable treatment options. Clinical trials accept patients even while receiving chemotherapy or radiation therapy. It is recommended that patients join clinical trials immediately after diagnosis.

Chapter Four: Complementary and Alternative Medicine

Some patients may want to discover the benefits and risks of alternative and complementary practices. Practitioners of alternative methods use specific therapies to replace conventional treatment. But doctors use complementary therapies alongside cancer treatment to help improve the outcomes. Examples of alternative practices are Chinese medicine, osteopathic medicine, diet and herbs, and many others. Scientists and researchers cannot prove the effectiveness of alternative methods but have discovered that a few complementary practices such as acupuncture, yoga, and meditation work well when joined with standard practices.

Although these methods don't offer a cure for cancer, they can help reduce the side effects of chemotherapy, radiation therapy, and surgery. Your oncologist won't tell you to use alternative therapies, but might recommend complementary approaches to go along or to use during or after completing treatment. Although several of these methods have worked for some people, it doesn't mean they will work for you. Your doctor's advice is vital should you consider using any of these approaches.

Chapter Five: Specialized Cancer Care

Doctors don't limit treatment to chemotherapy, radiation therapy, surgery, emotional counseling, and less-common forms such as hormonal therapy and immunotherapy. Along with continued primary care, your health-care team may introduce palliative care (at any phase of your survivorship) or hospice care (toward the end-of-life period), both as noncurative practices.

Doctors design these techniques to offer you the best quality of life during your survivorship. They comprise a skilled multidisciplinary team of professionals who work together in harmony to provide you with the most comfort. These types of specialized care also extend to helping caregivers, family members, and anyone within your environment to tackle the emotional stress.

They also help you control the many aspects of your life, including the costs of hospital stays, insurance, and preparing legal documents. Also, they offer bereavement services to help family members and friends cope with the loss of their loved ones after death. Palliative and hospice care services are available 24/7.

THE NEXT STEP

If you are a nonpatient, your most reasonable next step is to continue reading to learn how to stay that way. Knowing more about cancer enables you to take preventive measures to maintain good health. Knowledge can also arm you with tools to help patients who may be in desperate need.

If you are a newly diagnosed patient, regardless of the stage of your cancer, go to chapter two. Learn about the disease and risk factors. In subsequent chapters, you'll know how to pinpoint specific risk factors that may have contributed to causing your illness. Knowing specifics allows you to avoid potential future harm should your cancer become worse. Read chapters 3–5 and discover more resources about the embedded information; they are essential in directing you to make the right treatment plan with minimal side effects. They are also crucial to helping you choose a wellness plan to go along with the treatment you choose for added benefits.

Before you move to part two, the strategy, you must know your exact position on the continuum (this chapter). Knowing your correct position on the continuum (how bad your cancer is) will direct you to the specific chapter for your situation. For example, if you have just learned of your diagnosis, then the most rational course of action is to continue to chapter 6, "Understand Your Diagnosis." If you are in remission, either partial or complete, go to chapter 13, "Categorize Your Current Health in the Permanent Phase." At the end of the introduction to part two, I will summarize the strategy and the direction you should follow depending on your cancer situation at a given time. The summary allows you to see the whole survivorship journey from the top and makes the navigation easier.

CHAPTER TWO

CANCER FUNDAMENTALS

Cancer is the broad name for a multidisease system that encompasses over a hundred complex diseases that vary in their natures and response to treatment. Each cancer behavior is different from the others, and they all differ in their properties, origination, and treatment. All malignancies have two main features: they have uncontrolled cell growth, and they can spread to other areas of the human body. Each cancer type (breast, colon, lung, skin, etc.) is distinct. For example, although your cancer type maybe like someone else's, your cancer would still be different in the sense that treatment and side effects may differ depending on factors including your age, other diseases you may have, geographic location, and lifestyle habits.

Cancer is life-threatening and associated with a myriad of adverse psychological and physical issues. Figure 2:1, page 16, shows the horrifying collection of effects that may go with the illness. You may experience one or more of these effects depending on your type of cancer, stage, and on the treatment or a mix of treatments you have received. These effects are likely to change as you progress through the journey.

Your journey is unique. A range of states with varying degrees of intensities and impacts affect your experience. Cancer is composed of three states: the *developmental state*, observed through the emotional, physical, and mental effects because of the impact of diagnosis and treatment, the *socioeconomic state* which combines education and financial matters, and the *psychosocial support state*, comprised of mental health counseling, spiritual and cultural facets, and group support. Most cancer patients will experience all the three states during their journeys. Your cancer, personality, and the support you receive are deciding factors on the type of influence these states will have on you.

A List of Side Effects of Cancer Surgery, Chemotherapy, and Radiation Therapy

Pain	Headaches
Fatigue	Muscle pain
Appetite loss	Stomach pain
Swelling	Shooting pain
Numbness	Mouth and throat sores
Constipation	Nausea and vomiting
Delirium	Stiff neck
Diarrhea	Vision problems
Edema	Hearing problems
Memory loss	Hair loss
Changes in thinking	Trouble breathing
Skin and nail changes	Weakened immune system
Sleep problems	Bruising
Bleeding	Rashes
Blood clots	Changes in skin color
Drug reactions	Mouth sores
Infections	Anxiety
Slow recovery	Depression
Lymphedema	Early menopause
Organ Dysfunction	Low blood cell count
Dietary concerns	Digestive distress
Body image issues	Bone loss
Infertility	Scarring
Heart problems	Speech problems
Lung problems	Secondary cancers
Kidney problems	Cataracts
Liver problems	Dry mouth
Hypertension	Thyroid problems
Endocrine problems	Self-esteem problems
Digestive problems	Financial distress
Psychological problems	Communication difficulty
Urinary and bladder problems	Weight gain and loss
Neuropathy	Lactose intolerance
Osteoporosis	Changes in taste and smell
Gas and bloating	And a few more

Figure 2:1. Effects of standard cancer treatments.

This dread disease has become a household name, a despised infiltrator capable of toppling your family's life with vigor. It can destroy you without scrutinizing how wealthy or how loving of an individual you are. It illustrates a concise, non-discriminatory protocol in action, successful in every way.

This chapter offers the essential knowledge you need to help you understand and progress through stages of the cancer continuum. It's best if you try to learn your diagnosis, your cancer's origin, risk factors, progression, staging, and treatment options. This knowledge is crucial to understanding your diagnosis.

DEFINITION

Several checkpoints in the human body prevent the uncontrolled proliferation of cells. Healthy cells commit suicide when they cannot pass various quality control tests; a built-in counting mechanism which reduces unnecessary cell divisions by imposing a limit on how many times a cell can divide; rigidity and physical partitions in tissues prevent the abnormal cellular clones from expanding. This genius regulation allows for cell balance in the human body, enabling only cells needed for specific duties to stay alive.

When healthy cells become abnormal, the results are cancer that evades the body's natural defenses and may spread (metastasize) to other parts of the body. There are several ways to delineate cancer, but I will define it in its purest form possible. It's a cluster of disorderly cells that divert from their natural assigned duties and performed unassigned functions. They stop obeying orders from the brain and, as a result, cease replenishment and continue to multiply through cell division and become out of control without following the rules necessary to give your body a healthy life. And they travel to other locations in the body and either settle in the new place or keep on moving to another nearby site, causing a trail of destruction. They crowd healthy cells and consume their food, leaving them, the healthy ones, craving for nutrients necessary to support their specified active duties.

Human cells must replenish themselves to allow new cells to take their place and sustain the development phases of life. Replenishment comes in the form of cell death when they stop playing a vital role. If those aging cells don't die, then we have a buildup of more cells. They carry the same damaged DNA as the mother cell, causing a problem when new cells are born while the old ones are still alive. Accumulation of the cells that did not die compile to form a tissue mass and form a lump or a tumor. Those are the cells that can create a path of destruction when they spread through the bloodstream or lymphatic system.

Sometimes, those cells are unstoppable to an extent. Different cancers are alike only in the definition; several are fast-growing; others grow at slower rates. Their response to treatment differs to where sometimes surgery is the best choice, but others respond better to chemotherapy or radiation therapy. Sometimes, a mix of treatments is needed to get the sought-after results.

Cancer can form at any location in the body. For example, in the lungs, breast, colon, or even in the blood. It's benign when non-life-threatening, the tumor is engulfed and not cancerous, or it occupies a specific location. Benign tumors don't metastasize. They don't spread or invade other parts of the body. Surgery is the primary procedure to remove most benign tumors, or doctors could leave them alone if they are not causing an issue such as pushing on nearby organs and causing pain. When doctors use surgery to remove the tumors, they make sure they won't grow back. Benign tumors start as a lump, such as in the breast.

Malignant tumors are the exact opposite. They are cancerous and can move to other areas of the body and either settle in the new location or keep on moving to infect a new site. They metastasize and invade nearby tissues and lymph nodes. Surgery can remove part of them, and doctors could shrink them in size through chemotherapy and radiation therapy, but they may come back. Malignant tumors can be fatal if they are aggressive in their advanced stages.

Some familiar words you might hear when describing cancer are *tumor*, *malignancy*, *neoplasm*, and *lesion*. Although we can use all those words interchangeably, they have different definitions. The medical community defines neoplasm as an overgrowth of cells or any abnormal growth; it could be benign or malignant such as in skin cancers. A lesion means an unusual spot usually caused by injury or disease. Doctors may refer to benign or malignant mouth ulcers and bruises of the arms as lesions; they are bumps on the skin in little blemishes of cancer. [R15]

TYPES OF CANCERS

Carcinoma: Cancer that starts in the epithelial tissue of the skin or the lining of internal organs. Examples of carcinoma include breast, lung, and colon cancers. Carcinomas cover and line the organs—for example, the organs of the digestive system. And they line the body cavities, such as the inside of the chest and the abdominal cavities. Carcinoma further is comprised of subgroups, including squamous cell carcinoma found in the area such as the skin or the lining of the throat or esophagus. Adenocarcinoma starts in the glandular cells (found in the cervix and the lining of the uterus). Transitional cell carcinoma is a type of cancer that begins in the bladder's lining. These cells can stretch as the organ expands.

Sarcoma: Cancer that starts in the bone, cartilage, fat, muscle, blood vessels, or other connective supportive tissue. It arises from transformed cells of mesenchymal (the connective tissue found during the embryo's development) origin. Human sarcomas are rare.

Leukemia: Cancer of the body's blood-forming tissues, including the bone marrow and the lymphatic system. Leukemia is cancer of the blood. When the white blood cells produced in the bone marrow are disrupted, they become cancerous. White blood cells are potent infection fighters. They resemble other healthy cells in the body. They divide and grow in a fashion as needed. Leukemia can take on many forms, a few are common in children, but it also exists in adults.

Lymphoma and multiple myeloma: Both types of these cancers occur when cancer targets the cells that are components of the white blood cells. Since the bone marrow is the leading factory to produce cells, it becomes an easy target for the growth of abnormal plasma cells. As the name shows, lymphomas are cancers of the lymphatic system. They target lymphocytes, which play an essential role in the immune system. Hodgkin and non-Hodgkin are the most common forms of lymphoma. We cannot prevent lymphoma, although survival rates after treatment are excellent. Myeloma is also a cancer of the plasma cells. Multiple myelomas denote more than one myeloma, and permanent remedy is available. Both lymphoma and myeloma begin in the cells of the immune system.

Central nervous system cancer: Lymphoma that targets the brain and the spinal cord, the central nervous system (CNS), where the cancer cells form in the lymph tissue of the brain or the spinal cord. A weakened immune system is a trap for increasing the risk of developing primary CNS lymphoma.

The site of its origination names the cancer in question. For example, when it starts in the breast, doctors call it breast cancer. Even if it spreads to another location of the body, it's still cancer of the breast. [R16]

CANCER CAUSES

Although our bodies are made up of billions of cells, cancer starts in only one of those cells when it loses control of cell division or cellular death. This single, disturbed cell gives rise to other cells that may appear in certain parts of the body. This process isn't instant; it may take months or even years after the initial disruption of the single cell.

Something must trigger the first cell to become disobedient! For cells to grow abruptly, they must have been under undesirable pressure that made them snap and become disruptive. Doctors offer plenty of cancer risk factors (something that increases the chance of developing a disease) that may trigger the cells to mutate and become cancerous.

Cell mutation is a well-known cause of cancer. When changes occur in the genes that are part of the DNA, they order cells to either divide too quickly or prevent them from dying. In either case, the result is a pile of mutated cells that have no specific purpose in the body. Mutations can be inherited or caused by external factors such as viruses, chemicals, or physical agents. Mutation does not always mean cancer; the cell may have to gain a second or even a third mutation to become cancerous, and it may also never happen. Exposure to carcinogens does not always produce cancer in everyone. It depends on how quickly your body converts these chemicals and how much is converted by the body into harmless substances. Some people may not be affected by carcinogens in their entire life. People handle cancer-causing agents differently.

Carcinogens (a substance capable of triggering the disease in living tissue) can result from your lifestyle habits—for example, smoking—or can be factors imposed on you by the environment, such as harmful rays from the sun. Sometimes an escape from environmental factors isn't possible, but there is always an escape from negative lifestyle habits. There is still something you can do to reduce your exposure to cancer-causing agents.

Digging into risk factors that may have contributed to your condition won't cure your cancer, but it will help you to better self-manage your survivorship. This knowledge will teach you how to avoid certain lifestyle habits to lessen the effects of treatment and reduce the chances of cancer recurrence or even developing second cancers. [R17]

TREATMENT OPTIONS

The progressiveness of your cancer determines the most suitable treatment for you. Knowledge of your cancer treatment options and their side effects will help you decide on the most viable therapy.

Sometimes you don't have many treatment choices. But other times, you may have multiple options depending on your situation. In certain circumstances, a mix of different treatments is necessary, such as combining surgery with chemotherapy or radiation therapy. Others could be immunotherapy, targeted therapy, hormone therapy, or a few others.[R18] clinical trials (chapter 3) and complementary therapies (chapter 4) are choices to consider alongside with your treatment for a possibility of improving the outcomes and for lessening the side effects. Take into consideration the undesirable side effects when you decide on the most suitable treatment and how they may affect your life. There are many treatments available:

Surgery

Surgery is the removal of a malignant mass and is executed through making use of small, thin knives called *scalpels* to cut through the skin, muscles, and sometimes the bone. Your doctor will apply anesthesia (local, regional, or general) depending on the kind and location of the surgery performed.

According to MD Anderson Cancer Center, about 60 percent of patients will undergo some surgery to treat their cancer. Surgery could be the only necessary form of therapy doctors use for specific situations. There are many types of cancer surgery, serving various purposes. Some of these types are listed below.

Diagnostic surgery, also called a *surgical biopsy*, is a small cut, called an *incision*, made to the skin to remove some or all of the suspicious tissue. An *incisional biopsy* is used to remove only a piece of the suspected area, and an *excisional biopsy* is used to altogether eliminate the tumor (for example, a mole or a lump). The pathologist (the doctor who tests the extracted sample) examines the tissue and gives his or her findings to your oncologist in the pathology report.

Staging surgery determines the extent of cancer (how bad it is). It finds out the size of the tumor and where cancer has spread. Doctors perform this surgery by using an endoscope to view the suspicious area and take a tissue sample; an incision is unnecessary in this case. The doctor often also removes some lymph nodes near the tumor to find out if it has spread. Information from such a procedure can help predict a person's prognosis and may also be included in the pathology report.

Curative Surgery is the removal of the whole cancerous tumor and is followed by chemotherapy or radiation therapy to ensure the removal of all the cancerous cells. Doctors use this surgery for localized cancers that have not spread to nearby locations in the body.

Debulking is used for hard-to-reach locations of cancer or when its removal might harm the body. When it isn't workable for the surgeon to eliminate the whole tumor in a particular area, he or she tries to remove as much of it as possible. Usually, this procedure is followed by radiation or chemotherapy to continue treating the cancer and can also be given before surgery to help reduce the size of the tumor so the surgeon can remove it.

Palliation or palliative surgery is to relieve the pain of some side effects caused by cancer. Pressure on a nerve, spinal cord, bowel, an intestinal-tract obstruction, or any constraint on any part of the body can cause pain. Doctors also use palliative surgery to help stop bleeding caused by certain cancers such as in the areas with large amounts of blood vessels as in the case of the uterus, or in delicate organs that easily bleed when food and waste products pass through, such as the esophagus, stomach, and bowel. Various other advantages of palliative surgery include preventing breakage of weakened bone because of cancer treatment. This procedure is done by inserting a metal rod to help stop the splitting and breaking of weak bones, and these rods stay in place for the entire healing process.

Reconstruction surgery is cosmetically repairing a cancer site after surgery. Doctors can perform this surgery concurrently with the primary cancer surgery or a while after they complete the procedure. It's used to restore the body's appearance or function. An example of reconstructive surgeries is breast reconstruction after a mastectomy.

Prevention surgery is often used to lower the risk of getting cancer and stop it from occurring, such as with removing colon polyps before they become malignant. Or, when some women have the breast removed (*mastectomy*) or the ovaries removed (*oophorectomy*) if they have a strong family history of breast or ovarian cancers. Having these types of surgeries done will reduce the risk of getting breast or ovarian cancers.

Not all cancer surgeries involve cutting deep through the skin. There is minimally invasive surgery, also called *keyhole* or *laparoscopic surgery*, that uses advanced techniques to remove the tumor through tiny incisions. It can also be performed through robotic arms controlled by the surgeon. Minimally invasive surgery inflicts minimal pain, and the body heals faster than the conventional method. These surgeries have a smaller impact on the patient. They cause less blood loss and decreased need for blood transfusion, shorter hospital stays, less pain, fewer pain medications, quicker recovery, and less scarring. These procedures aren't suitable for many cancer surgeries.

Radiation Therapy

Radiation therapy, also called *radiotherapy*, uses high doses of radiation (X-rays, gamma rays, or electrons) directed at the cancerous mass to kill the cells and shrink tumors. It's also used to lessen the pain in patients, and it can cure certain types of cancers. Doctors use the high doses to kill the cancerous cells or shrink their growth by damaging their DNA beyond repair. When damage occurs to the DNA, it causes cell death. The body removes the dead cells after they further break down. This process does not happen during the radiation session; it may take days or weeks of treatment before damaging the DNA enough for cancer cells to die. The cancer cells continue to die for weeks or months after radiation therapy ends. Radiation differs from chemo in the sense that it's localized; it only affects the irradiated area in the body. The result is less damaging to healthy tissues, leading to fewer side effects. Receiving radiation can be external for the patient, such as aiming a high energy beam at certain spots of cancer. Doctors also administer radiotherapy by injecting a radioactive source in the mouth, or it can be delivered through inserting "seeds" of radiation in or near the tumor (*brachytherapy*).

Chemotherapy

Chemotherapy is a treatment that uses potent drugs to kill cancerous cells and is considered the most common procedure. It uses chemicals to treat disease. All chemical medicines to treat any disease are chemotherapy. Chemotherapy comes as a pill that you could take orally or inject in your vein or muscle. Sometimes, doctors may have to pump the medicine directly into spinal fluids, or into the artery or another part of the body. The method of receiving drugs depends on the cancer and the health requirements of the patient. When the cancerous cells are not reachable through surgery or radiation therapy, then chemotherapy would be the best option. It's systemic, meaning it treats the entire system or body. Chemotherapy drugs kill healthy cells in their path, causing unwanted side effects, and they can be mild or rough.

Chemotherapy works like radiotherapy through causing cell death or through slowing cell growth. Chemotherapy can cure cancer at early stages, lessen the chances of recurrence, or shrink tumors that are causing pain and other problems.

Immunotherapy

Immunotherapy, or *biological therapy,* is a treatment that strengthens the immune system and enables it to fight cancer; it stimulates the body's immune system. The immune system aids your body to fight infections and other diseases. It is comprised of white blood cells, organs, and tissues of the lymph system. It uses substances made from living organisms to treat cancer. One way cancer cells thrive is through hiding from the immune system. Some immunotherapies mark these cells to help your immune system to find and destroy them.

There are several types of immunotherapy that help the immune system act against cancer, including checkpoint inhibitors, adoptive cell transfer, monoclonal antibodies, and treatment vaccines. It's a new approach that is becoming a part of standard therapy for some cancers but remains investigational for other types. Usually, immunotherapy is administered intravenously (IV) and goes into the vein, orally through pills or capsules, topically through a cream that you can rub on your skin (cannot be used for skin cancer), or intravesical, which means immunotherapy goes directly into the bladder.

As with almost all cancer therapies, immunotherapy can cause side effects depending on factors such as the type of cancer, stage, how healthy you were before cancer treatment, the therapy you are receiving, and the dose. Side effects of this therapy vary for different individuals, but you may experience some mild or severe side effects such as pain, redness, itching, soreness, fever, fatigue, dizziness, nausea, headaches, trouble breathing, swelling, or risk of infection.

You may receive immunotherapy every day, weekly, or monthly depending on cancer, type of immunotherapy you receive, and how your body reacts to the treatment. It's administered in cycles (periods) to give your body the chance to rest and heal.

Targeted Therapy

This treatment aims at the changes in cancer cells that help them grow (divide). It's the basis of precision medicine. Although this therapy uses drugs, it differs from traditional chemotherapy. The National Cancer Institute (NCI) explains that the difference between the two is that targeted therapy acts on specific molecular targets that are associated with cancer, whereas most standard chemotherapies act on all rapidly dividing healthy and cancerous cells. Targeted therapies are deliberately chosen to interact with their target, whereas many conventional chemotherapies were identified because they kill cells. They are often cytostatic (they block cell proliferation), whereas traditional chemotherapy agents are cytotoxic (they kill tumor cells).

Targeted therapy targets specific genes, proteins, or the tissue environment (found in cancer cells) that contribute to cancer growth and progression and spread of cancer. It enables researchers to design better, promising therapies that target these changes or block their effect.

Targeted therapy is less toxic than traditional chemotherapy because cancer cells are more dependent on the target than on healthy cells. Targeted therapies act on specific molecular targets that are associated with cancer; they interact with their targets. On the contrary, chemotherapy acts on all rapidly dividing normal and cancerous cells— they are identified because they kill cells.

However, targeted therapies *can* also have side effects including diarrhea, skin rashes, nail changes, blood clotting, hair depigmentation, liver problems such as hepatitis and elevated liver enzymes, gastrointestinal perforation (ruptured bowel, a hole in the wall of part of the gastrointestinal tract), slow wound healing time, and high blood pressure. The severity of side effects differs for different patients and mainly depends on their health before the treatment.

Hormone Therapy

Hormone therapy is a treatment that slows or stops the growth of cancers that use hormones to grow, such as in the breast and prostate. Specialists use this method to lessen the chance that cancer will return, slow it, and even stop its growth. For men with prostate cancer unable to use surgery or radiation therapy to reduce or prevent symptoms, then hormonal therapy may be a suitable choice.

When hormone therapy is used with other forms of treatment, it can shrink the tumor before surgery or radiation therapy. This treatment is called *neoadjuvant therapy*. It can also lower the risk of cancer recurrence after primary treatment, called *adjuvant therapy*. Also, it can destroy cells that have returned or spread to other parts of the body.

As with almost all cancer treatments, hormone therapy can have some unwanted side effects like those of targeted therapies. Some less-common side effects in women who receive this treatment to treat breast cancer include hot flashes, vaginal dryness, changes in period, and mood changes, along with nausea, fatigue, and vomiting.

Stem Cell Transplant

Also called a *bone marrow transplant*. Patients who need their blood-forming stem cells restored after being destroyed by high doses of chemo or radiation can use this type of therapy. There are three types of stem cell transplants:

- o Autologous is when the stem cells come from you, the patient.
- o Allogeneic is when the stem cells come from someone else. The donor may be a blood relative or someone not related to you.
- o Syngeneic is when the stem cells come from your identical twin, if you have one.

To reduce the side effects and improve the chances that the transplant will work, the donor's blood-forming stem cells must match yours in specific ways.

Stem cell transplants rarely affect cancer cells in a straight manner. Instead, they help recover your ability to produce stem cells after treatment with high doses of radiation, chemotherapy, or both. There are a few circumstances where stem cells may work straight against cancer cells, as with multiple myeloma and some types of leukemia. This result happens because of an effect called *graft-versus-tumor* that can take place after allogeneic transplants. Graft-versus-tumor takes place when leukocytes from your contributor (the graft) work against any cancer cells that remain in your body (the growth) after high-dose therapies. This effect boosts the success of the treatment.

You cannot escape specific side effects because of stem cell transplant. Since you'll receive chemotherapy with or without radiation before the stem cell transplant, many of these treatment side effects will resemble chemotherapy and radiation therapy effects. The most severe side effect is the high risk of infection from low levels of white blood cells.

Other possible immediate side effects include mouth sores, fatigue, diarrhea, nausea, vomiting, low level of platelets (which can decrease how well blood can clot), and anemia (low levels of red blood cells). Long-term side effects may include infertility, cataracts, early menopause, thyroid issues, lung or bone damage, and risk of developing another cancer.

Precision Medicine

Precision medicine is a method that includes treatments of your cancer based on genetic understanding. Doctors call it *personalized medicine* and hope to tailor it to the genetic changes in each person's cancer. This concept isn't new, but advances in medicine and technology have helped speed up research in this area of disease treatment. Precision medicine is a promising field in cancer treatment, and it's beyond this book.

For further readings on the various treatment, refer to the general resources section. Or, for specific treatment methods, refer to R18.

CANCER STAGING

Staging is a measure of cancer spread in the body to help doctors know its severity and the chances of survival, along with determining the most suitable treatment options. It enables you to discover various other opportunities that may help with the treatment, such as clinical trials or complementary and alternative therapies (chapters 3 and 4).

Staging is one process during your diagnosis that provides the most information on your cancer. The stage does not change, regardless of changes in your condition. The new information on how the cancer has changed gets added to the original information. Various types of tests and medical procedures, such as x-rays or lab tests, can find the stage.

When the stage is known, you can find a large amount of information on your cancer at that stage. For example, the tumor's location in the body, cell types (for example, adenocarcinoma or squamous cell carcinoma), size, whether it has metastasized to other parts of the body or nearby lymph nodes, and the tumor grade. The stage also refers to cell abnormality and how likely the tumor to grow and travel to other sites of the body. There are various staging systems:

The TNM Staging System

This system is the most-used method for most cancers. Brain or spinal cord tumors may use different staging systems. The TNM staging system is what you'll find on your pathology report, and it's the primary cancer-reporting system.

In the TNM system, T refers to the size and extent of the primary tumor, N refers to the number of nearby lymph nodes that contain cancer, and the M refers to if cancer has metastasized.

When using the TNM system, the numbers after each letter give more details on cancer. The following example explains the combinations of letters and numbers in T1N0MX or T3N1M0.

Primary tumor (T):

- TX: The primary tumor isn't measurable.
- T0: The primary tumor is absent.
- T1, T2, T3, T4: The numbers refer to the size and how far cancer has traveled.

T describes the size of the tumor. The higher the number after the T, the larger it is. It could show how far it has matured into nearby tissues. We may further divide the Ts to get more detail, such as T3a and T3b.

Regional lymph nodes (N):

- NX: The X shows that lymph nodes are not measurable.
- N0: Cancer is absent in nearby lymph nodes.
- N1, N2, N3: The numbers after the N refer to the number of lymph nodes that contain cancer. The higher the number, the higher the number of lymph nodes containing cancer.

Distant metastasis (M):

- MX: The X shows that metastasis isn't measurable.
- M0: A sign that cancer has not spread; it's localized.
- M1: Cancer has metastasized to other parts of the body.

Doctors can interpret the TNM staging system with fewer details, making it simple for the layman to understand. There are other staging systems used by doctors for specific processes, including:

- Stage 0: Shows abnormal cells, but they have not spread to nearby tissue. Another name is *in situ*.
- Stage I, II, III: Cancer is present. The higher the number, the larger the tumor and the extent of spread into nearby tissues.
- Stage IV: Cancer has spread to other parts of the body, metastasized.

SYMPTOMS OF CANCER

Cancer, being a multidisease system, can cause many symptoms of various types. Symptoms depend on the type and size of cancer, whether it had metastasized, and how much it's affected its surrounding organs or tissues. If cancer spreads to other parts of the body, then the symptoms and signs may appear in different areas, not only the original location.

Doctors associate the following seven symptoms with cancer and summarize them in one easy-to-remember word: CAUTION. Each letter in the word shows the first letter of a sign.

- Changes in bowel or bladder habits
- A sore that does not heal
- Unusual bleeding or discharge
- Thickening or a lump in the breast, including changes in the nipple size or shape and variations in the texture of the breast skin or any other part of the body
- Indigestion or problems swallowing
- Obvious change in a wart or mole
- Nagging cough or hoarseness

The above symptoms alert you of general indications that cancer may exist, but the list isn't comprehensive. Other symptoms and signs may appear, such as discomfort after eating, hard time swallowing, and changes in appetite when there are no reasons for weight gain or loss. Abdominal pain accompanied by unexplained night sweats and feeling weak or exhausted can serve as signs that something is wrong.

Other less severe conditions may cause these symptoms, and they don't mean you have cancer. But having any of the symptoms above, you may have to visit your doctors for further testing.

If you have symptoms lasting for long periods, you need to see a doctor to perform a diagnosis and repair the problem as early as possible. Early cancers don't cause pain, so see your doctor before experiencing any symptoms or pain.

When cancer grows, it causes signs, symptoms, and sometimes pain because of pushing on nearby organs, nerves, and blood vessels. Sometimes, a small tumor can cause symptoms if it's present in sensitive parts and organs of the body, such as the brain.

Cancer will have to be large enough to cause signs and symptoms. For example, pancreatic tumors won't cause symptoms until they grow large enough to press on nearby nerves or organs, causing abdominal and back pain. Others may accumulate around the bile duct and cause a blockage of the bile flow, which in turn causes the eyes and the skin to appear yellow (jaundice). By the time these signs or symptoms emerge, cancer is in an advanced stage and has metastasized beyond the place of origin.

If cancer causes fever, extreme tiredness, or weight loss, then it may have used up the body's energy supply, or it may have released substances that change the way the body makes energy from food. Cancers can release contents into the bloodstream that causes specific symptoms. For example, certain pancreatic tumors can release substances that cause blood clots in the veins of the legs. Lung cancers make hormone-like substances that raise blood calcium levels, affecting nerves and muscles, making you feel weak, tired, and dizzy. The damage can also cause changes in how your immune system works.

Noticing cancer symptoms allows your doctor to detect cancer early and to find the problem as soon as possible to increase the chances of a solution. A great example is the early detection of melanoma; the five-year survival rate is around 98 percent if it's not grown deep into the skin, and this would be an instance of cancer not causing any symptoms until it has spread.

Doctors can detect certain tumors before they show any symptoms. The best way to spot these cancers before they produce any signs and symptoms is by having regular checkups and screening tests. It may or may not be cancer. If not cancer, your doctor will diagnose your condition and treat it. If it's cancer, you may have had the chance to have it detected early, as well as a high likelihood of a cure when the treatment works best.

Specialized tests are available for people with a family history of cancer. Exposure to specific risk factors may need specialized examinations. The need for specialized lab tests depends on your situation. There are circumstances where more aggressive testing is necessary.[R19]

THE FUTURE OF YOUR CANCER

Upon learning of your cancer diagnosis, many questions circulate in your head. You may want to know how bad your cancer is and whether it's getting worse. You might want to know about your chances of survival and inquire about the possibility of your cancer going into remission. Some patients abstain from gaining specific information about the future of their cancer since the answers are statistical and not definitive of their conditions.

Although you may feel discouraged to learn your disease outlook, it might help you further adjust to new health needs to get the hopeful results. Brief definitions of specific terms when describing the future of your cancer, including *progression*, *remission*, and *prognosis* are covered below.

Progression: Tumors change during their life and become more aggressive in their behaviors; they become more malignant, thus more dangerous. This phenomenon is called *tumor progression*; it happens toward the third and the last phase of cancer development. In this final phase, the tumor may gain higher malignant potentials. The National Cancer Institute defines progression as the course of a disease, such as cancer, as it becomes worse or spreads in the body. It's when cancer goes from bad to worse.

On the molecular level, the accumulation of genetic mutations gives rise to the phenomenon of progression. Genetic mutations result in the activation and inactivation of oncogenes and suppressor genes, giving advanced cancer the ability, at the cellular level, to evade the immune system, stimulate blood supply development, invade surrounding tissues, and metastasize. Observing progression happens when the cancer is symptomatic, which characterizes a late stage, making the study of this phenomenon difficult. Progression is the opposite of regression, which is when tumor shrinks in size or when it's disappearing.

Remission: Cancer can go into remission, either partial or complete, which means the signs and symptoms are reduced. In complete remission, signs or symptoms will disappear. If those signs and symptoms stay absent for five years or more, then you may consider yourself cured of cancer.

In some cases, cells may have remained in your body for an extended period after treatment, and your disease may come back. It's the reason you'll never hear your oncologist say you are free of cancer. They might declare you as cancer-free for now or might say, "There are no signs of the disease," hoping it never comes back.

When remission lasts for a long time, doctors call it durable remission. It isn't known how long it lasts, and it depends on many factors and characteristics of your cancer, such as type and stage. If the tumor disappears by itself without treatment, then doctors call it *spontaneous remission*. It's a rare event, but it can occur with many types of cancers. Spontaneous remission is a hope every cancer patient has, and it's possible with no apparent reason—more on this topic in later chapters.[R21]

Prognosis: This is a prediction about what will happen with your cancer. It's a guess made by your doctor based on numbers found from many past cancer cases sharing similarities with your cancer situation. The resulting numbers are not specific to your condition. They depend on the cancer, stage, progressiveness (how advanced it is), your age, your physical fitness, and whether you have any other health issues. A lot can happen during your journey to influence those numbers; sometimes, the impact can be decisive, where the same factors can have the opposite effects. Your prognosis information is vital for doctors since it helps them find the best treatment plan for you. Although prognosis numbers lack accuracy, they help to understand how dangerous your immediate and long-term situations are, and that allows everyone within your circle to prepare for the future.

Every cancer patient will have questions about their disease outlook. Learning about your prognosis may trigger an emotional moment that will most likely shape and alter your way of thinking about your cancer and yourself. Prognosis is a challenge to understand and difficult to speak about even with your doctor. Part of you wants to know it's an uphill battle.

Many factors affect your future outlook, such as your cancer stage, grade, traits of the cancer cells, your age, your health before cancer, and your response to treatment. Advances in cancer treatments make a precise prognosis even more challenging to produce. New, safer, and more effective treatments are becoming available, and you might be subjected to such treatments. When these new treatments become available to you, your prognosis might change and produce more favorable numbers.

During the prognosis discussion with your doctor, there will be many questions to ask. A few answers may confuse and frustrate you or even frighten you because of your state of denial. It might be best if you decide on how much information you want to absorb. Sometimes, learning more about your prognosis will give you the chance to improve your self-management skills and improve the outcomes. Remember that prognosis figures are only statistical and may not apply to your case. Try never to get discouraged by the numbers. They are only numbers to help your oncologist provide you with a *general* idea about your disease outlook.[R20]

When people get cancer, many questions circulate in their heads. Although to some people these queries may be irrational, it's actually the contrary. They are legitimate for the patient to inquire about. The most popular question is, "Why did I get cancer?"

WHY NOT EVERYONE GETS CANCER

I will conclude this chapter by providing you with a brief statement about why not everyone gets cancer. The shock you may have experienced during your diagnosis meeting with your oncologist might have given rise to this question and a multitude of others. To answer this question, we must have an idea about the causes of the disease. The medical community is unsuccessful in pinpointing the exact causes of cancer. They cannot understand the precise triggers because of the many variables that contribute to the complexity of the disease, but they know the risk factors that can cause cancer.

Certain risk factors including age, gender, and family history are beyond our control. But we can control a few important risk factors related to our lifestyles, including smoking, alcohol consumption, obesity, exposure to carcinogens, and other environmental factors.

To respond to such questions, we must consider that exposure to environmental factors (carcinogens), given over the same period, may affect people differently depending on the strength of their immunity. Carcinogenic exposure may have no impact on individuals with a healthy immune system, while it may have adverse effects on individuals with compromised (weak) defenses.

The following example illustrates variance in immunity. Two individuals are in a small, enclosed space, subjected to the same microorganism, such as the cold virus. One with a healthy immune system resists it and stay cold-free, while the other individual with a weak immune system gets the virus.

The same applies to cancer when infection, illness, lifestyle habits, and various medications play a role in compromising your immunity. Your immune system is your primary defense mechanism against external and internal factors that may harm your body. With cancer, your susceptibility to disease increases and your defenses become deficient. Developing cancer isn't your fault, although you may have played a small role in triggering the disease. For now, it suffices to say cancer and other diseases affect people depending on a multitude of factors. Some people's resistance to disease is higher than others for various reasons where genetic factors can play a significant role. ^{R22}

CHAPTER THREE

CLINICAL TRIALS

Doctors and medical researchers can offer you a chance to try new medicines and future therapies today. Some people may have reservations about the above words and perceive them as sarcastic. Others take advantage of this research just because it gives them hope. You may not agree with clinical trials because doctors cannot determine the accuracy and validity of the results, but others might welcome the idea.

Even though the new study may not help one situation, it may help others. A friend of mine who had an aggressive metastatic cancer said, "What do I have to lose? I'm dying anyway, and clinical trials are my only glimpse of hope of living an extra day."

You shouldn't take my friend's words as a standard measure in making your decision to join. For some people, clinical trials prove beneficial at any stage of their cancer.

I will introduce you to the science of cancer clinical trials, and the decision to join or abstain is yours to make. It may be an option you want to consider depending on your situation. You may take part because you want to try a new drug or treatment for your illness. Alternatively, you might do it because it helps doctors develop better therapies for the future that may benefit other patients.

This chapter defines clinical trials and their phases. It advises you of the benefits and risks involved and your eligibility to join but pursue other credible avenues to collect vital information about your specific case. Your starting point in the collection process begins by consulting your oncologist. Contacting the National Clinical Trials Network (NCTN) and the National Cancer Institute is also a good way to start your search for a suitable clinical trial for your cancer.

DEFINITION

When a new drug or treatment, performed on lab animals, shows antitumor tendencies, then it's studied in humans. When researchers prove these investigational drugs safe and effective, they become a part of standard treatment. Doctors, lab technicians, and scientists from various disciplines who are professionals in a medical subject (such as cancer) perform such studies. They involve research with new, experimental treatments and the different ways to use them.

These types of studies include people willing to take part in the trials. It's a lengthy process that may take years before completion. Before using any new treatment on patients, scientists work for long years to understand the disease under study. They arrange studies to investigate new treatment and side effects on humans and lab animals. Doctors can offer this cancer research when the FDA approves it as a new treatment for certain cancers.

Clinical trials are comprised of four different goals: search for new treatments, learn the side effects and symptoms of a disease like cancer, investigate long-term side effects of treatment, and prevent and look for cancer. Trials can offer you financial relief since they provide treatment and follow-up at no cost to you, but certain cost restrictions can apply when you live a far distance from the trial base.

Nowadays, people are living longer and enjoying a good quality of life after successful therapies because of past trials. Attendance is a voluntary process, but when you join, no one forces you to complete all the phases. You can leave whenever you want.

You can attend a clinical trial no matter the type or stage of your cancer. Your admission is possible even if you have aggressive cancer that isn't responding to treatment. Doctors encourage patients living with advanced diseases to take a role in clinical trials to possibly improve their prognosis. Sometimes, aggressive cancers may trigger stress, making patients less able to comprehend simple data related to their cancer. In these situations, the health-care team will explain the information in a form the patient can understand.

It's a reasonable option for you to attend a trial if your present standard treatment isn't useful anymore and your doctor thinks it may help to join. Patients whose cancers are less severe may look at it to complement their current treatment or to control side effects.

In the United States, testing new drugs through clinical trials is a base requirement for approval by the FDA. The approval process is a requirement to ensure the safety of all present and future cancer patients.

Several clinical trials that investigate a drug or treatment can happen concurrently. Multiple tests are necessary since doctors are always looking for new information and new treatment therapies with reduced side effects. They are supervised and run by reputable cancer organizations, including the National Cancer Institute, through cooperative groups of oncologists.

Can clinical trials help cancer? They might. Clinical trials offer much hope for many people with cancer when the standard approaches are no longer useful. You may receive a treatment that provides you with the best chance for doing well. Most times, you may receive a new, experimental drug before the authorities approve it, and it may work for you.

If you join, you'll get the same level of care you would with cancer treatment at the hospital or clinic. Your health-care team will monitor your health needs and offer you the best care while at the trial. They will help you improve your quality of life during and after treatment. Future patients can enjoy the positive results and knowledge gathered from such studies.

Sometimes, clinical trials may include lots of patients waiting in line to get in—numbers could be in the hundreds or thousands—leading to delayed results.

If a clinical trial accepts you as a patient, your oncology and lab team will explain all the steps before you begin. They will answer all your questions with the highest accuracy. They will help you make the critical decision about joining and do everything they can to make your time worthwhile and beneficial.

THE PHASES OF TRIALS

Clinical trials are comprised of phases; each has distinct characteristics and requirements. They designate time intervals for patients to go through for the duration of a clinical trial. They are phases 0, I, II, III, and IV, written in Roman numerals. All clinical trials must start with phase 0 or I. Phases contain different information about the treatment being studied, giving doctors the data about the drug they intend to explore. The main phases are I, II, and III.

Phase 0 studies are exploratory and differ from all other phases. Phase 0 is a routine phase to help speed up and streamline the drug approval process. In this phase, doctors use small doses of the new drug. Unlike the others, phase 0 has no benefit to the patient. Since the doses given to the patient are low, there is no risk that the patient develops side effects.

In this phase, doctors try to discover whether the drug reaches the tumor and the many consequences resulting from administering the medication and how the body responds to it, if it does. Before the patient receives the new drug, they undergo various medical tests that may include biopsies, scans, and blood samples. Researchers hope to find out more information about the drug and if it meets its intended purpose.

Any slight problems with the way the patient absorbs the drug or how it acts in the body should become apparent at this stage. If the drug does not produce the sought-after result, the researcher will stop such a study, which reduces cost and saves time. The number of people involved in this phase is fewer than fifteen.

Phase I focuses on the drug rather than the patient. It serves the advanced science of oncology more than anything else. Once doctors get the approval to use the medicine for human studies, they determine the optimal safe dose through testing such drugs in a small trial. This phase does not focus on improving the survival of an individual. Most likely, the patient won't understand his or her involvement in such a phase since there will be no benefit to them.

Phase I studies often involve patients with different cancers. They are for testing new drugs, and there is almost no data to present to the patient about expected results. The purpose is to concentrate on toxicity (the degree to which a particular substance can harm a human or an animal) and the starting dose rather than the patient. The aim is to discover a safe dosage, and when they find it, they decide on the method of how to administer it for a new treatment, its effects on the body, and its role in fighting cancer.

The number of patients wanting to take part (response rate) in phase I has always been low, but increased by a small margin since the focus was on the biology of the tumor and the pharmacology of the drug under consideration. The number of people taking part in this phase ranges from fifteen to thirty.

Phase II begins after testing the drug and proving its safety upon giving it to the patient. This phase examines the drug to find out if it's working on one or more specific types and stages of cancer. The results allow the oncologist to provide an early assessment of whether the drug works. The purpose is to decide if a drug influences specific cancer and to see how it affects the human body. It determines how it fights cancer, if it does. The number of people taking part in this phase is less than a hundred.

Phase III shows the result on the patient due to administering the drug. Phase III studies are more extensive studies that may involve hundreds or even thousands of patients depending on the facility's location—the concentration is on patients with specific types of cancers. Many phase III trials are randomized, meaning that researchers randomly pick patients who registered for the trial to receive the new treatment. The design of these trials intends to provide definitive evidence to support FDA approval of the drug or agent for public use. Phase III compares the new findings with the standard treatment to find distinctions and variations between them. The number of people taking part in this phase range in the hundreds, even thousands.

Phase IV is the follow-up period, taking place after approval of the drug and often called *post-marketing trials*. The goal is to ensure no safety or other concerns come up after the drug approval, and the pre-approval trials were error-free. Following patients for several years for observational purposes is essential. This allows doctors to determine any long-term side effects or other issues that the use of this drug may impose.

Clinical trials become seamless when researchers combine two phases, like I and II or II and III. The combinations allow for a smooth transition between phases and enable researchers to answer questions more quickly.

Each trial has a principal investigator, a doctor who prepares the plan for you. Another name for the procedure is *protocol*, and it contains needed information that helps the doctor decide if this treatment is right for you and what he or she needs to do. It also includes information concerning the reason for doing the trial and the eligibility criteria.

YOUR SAFETY AND OTHER ISSUES

At the start of a clinical trial, the staff will answer all your questions and review all the trial's information and offer guidance about the admission process to help you make your choice for joining.

During the clinical trial, the research staff will monitor your health and tell you about the medical tests and procedures you'll need to get done. After the clinical trial ends, the staff may check on you for several weeks, months, or even longer. They monitor you to ensure the treatment does not cause problems and determine how long it might work.

If you seek to join clinical trials, you must understand the benefits and the risks. It's your decision, so learning the positive and negative outcomes is an excellent foundation for you to make your choices.

Some benefits include accessing new treatments not available to everyone yet. Since you'll be under careful and close supervision, you'll enjoy more advanced and more effective treatments and help scientists progress to helping others through your contribution.

Risks include the possibility that a new treatment may not be better than the standard one and may carry unexpected side effects. Risks are not known ahead of time; there can be unexpected dangers. Doctors cannot predict future success, and they have less experience working with investigational drugs and treatments. You may have to make more visits to your doctor compared to when you were receiving the standard therapy. These additional visits may include an additional expense on you, including the possibility of travel, lodging, childcare at home, and loss of money due to missing work. Your doctor may also require more tests that could take up a lot of your time, and they may be uncomfortable.

You must understand that, since people are different, the treatment may not work for you even if it's working for someone else. Also, having other health problems besides cancer may complicate the issue, making the treatment offered by a clinical trial not work for you. To ensure that this problem does not arise, you'll receive medical tests to assess if you are fit for the trial.

Your insurance may not cover clinical research trials such as the study drug, lab test specific to your case, and any additional x-ray testing performed for your unique situation. Ask questions about the costs before you make your decision to join. Know your rights, financial matters, third-party sponsors, if any, changes in your daily life, job, and family issues. Let the doctor offer you a comparison between the old and the new treatments. If you take part in clinical trials, there are strict guidelines imposed by the federal government to ensure maximum safety for all participants. You should be aware of the following:

The stress involved: Trials may add to your emotional problems since you don't know what type of treatment or drugs you are receiving. Not knowing is a mystery that only adds to the list of your worries, hence elevating the pressures already imposed on you. Inform your health-care team of any changes in your emotional state during a trial and seek proper counseling.

The trial: Inquire about the purpose, length, possible outcomes, and who will oversee your care. Tell your trial team members about your concerns on the tests and treatments involved. Learn why they may think the new treatment may be better than the old one.

Risks and benefits: Ensure that your trial team provides and explains to you the risks and benefits in a language you can understand. Get information about past trials performed on other patients and compare the results. When the benefits outweigh the risks, you may proceed.

Your rights and costs: Ask about your privacy and the consequences should you leave the trial at the time of your choosing. Contact your insurance company and inquire about coverage or if they cover only parts of the process. On certain occasions, the administrative staff can provide you with information about organizations that may provide financial help.

Eligibility criteria: Before admittance to a clinical trial, doctors will check your eligibility. There are stringent guidelines to follow included in the study (called the *inclusion and exclusion criteria*). Admission depends on various data, including your type of cancer, gender, age, other health issues, and the treatments you may be undergoing. Once you have all that information in your possession, locate a clinical trial and perform your investigation to ensure you fit their eligibility criteria. Your next step is to contact the study team.

Your team will perform a prescreening evaluation before you appear in front of your study doctor for a consultation to determine your eligibility. You must answer many questions on the phone and in-person during the interview. Gather as much information as you can about your situation before your eligibility determination appointments.

Even after you choose a study, contact your primary care physician and try to get a second—even a third opinion, if possible. There are two types of costs involved in any trial: routine care cost and research costs. Health insurance companies include the cost of routine care sometimes. Get the full details from your company before you attempt to start as to avoid any future hardship related to clinical trials.

The trial itself will be for all the research portions. A trial does not cover personal expenses, and they may be your responsibility. Sometimes, the trial will offer you financial help to include some of your expenses, but you must contact your care team to inquire about it. Each trial is distinct, where expenses and time spent differ significantly.

What happens if you don't qualify? Doctors have established another avenue to help patients who need to try a new, unapproved drug when they have exhausted all other therapies. Doctors call it *compassionate drug use*.

When the US Food and Drug Administration (FDA) has not approved certain drugs, doctors designate them for compassionate use and call them *investigational drugs*. They're available to patients who are taking part in a clinical trial. However, what happens if you cannot join a clinical trial for any reason?

Although the use of compassionate drugs is legal, people who use them must meet certain conditions. If a clinical trial does not approve a patient to use such medicine, there will be two ways he or she can proceed: through expanded access and single-patient access programs.

Expanded access programs take place when a company sponsors a drug in the late stages of drug development, such as phase III clinical trials. The company can offer an expanded access program (EAP) for patients who cannot join a clinical trial. To be eligible for the EAP program, you must qualify and meet the EAP's requirements. The FDA would approve such a drug if it showed that it works at least somewhat to treat cancer.

Patients who qualify for neither clinical trials nor the EAP program can reserve the right to use single-patient access. If everything else fails, the patient may try to apply for this unique program.

Usually, it's hard to find a patient who qualifies for neither clinical trials nor the EAP. If such a patient is in existence, then the patient's doctor starts the process by talking first to the company that supplies the drug. The doctor will ask if they can use the drug for the patient and inquire about the possibility of the company providing it.

If the company agrees, then the doctor works with the drug company to ask the FDA to approve the drug to use in one patient. The doctor then supplies the required information by the FDA about the patient. He or she also provides the intended plan for the treatment and a signed consent form from the patient. The FDA can approve the request rapidly if no complications arise through the process, such as missing sensitive information about the patient treatment plan.

The process is frustrating for patients and doctors. The biggest problem is often the difficulty in getting the drug. Drug companies have different policies and procedures, and there is no way to force a company to surrender a drug. The company may have a limited supply available for compassionate use, or they may want to save the drug for clinical trials for whatever reason. When companies produce new medicine for people not in clinical trials, manufacturing can be costly for the drug company, especially when the FDA may never approve such a drug.

Getting compassionate drugs is a lengthy, confusing, and frustrating process. Several programs regulate compassionate use, and each agency has its own sets of regulations about the use of such drugs. There is the FDA, advocacy groups and organizations, the drugmaker, and the insurance companies. Each group or agency can't interfere with the other agency's rules, which makes it harder to get the drug.

The biggest problem is the cost; these investigational drugs cost a lot of money since they're new, and money spent on the research behind manufacturing them is enormous. Another hurdle is the precise regulation and restrictions imposed on them by the government. Although some drug companies may offer the drugs for free for clinical trials, others charge for the unapproved drugs. Your health insurance might not cover the additional costs, such as the clinical cost of administering the new medication and monitoring your response. Commonly, insurance companies don't cover investigational drugs.

There may also still, despite these hurdles, be patients who are approved for compassionate drug use. Because the definite purpose isn't well-documented, there are no numbers or statistics on how often doctors ask for them, or who's doing it. There are always unanswered questions on how well these are working for patients.

The National Cancer Institute's guidelines concerning compassionate drug use dictate that they are for patients who meet all the following conditions:

- Standard treatment did not work
- Not eligible for any current clinical trial that is using the drug
- Lack of other treatment options
- Have specific cancer for which there is a reason to expect the investigational drug will help
- When the benefits outweigh the risks involved

What are your thoughts about clinical trials? The rational approach to any subject is to visualize the results. Since everyone hopes for the best in any situation, we must be able to know, sense, or at least feel what's ahead. In your specific case, it will be difficult to know whether a trial will produce hopeful results or nothing at all. But in extreme cancer situations, trying anything new may be rational.

The trial may have produced nothing of value in your case, but the results may be valuable for the future of cancer. Success is a win situation for you and all others who need such gain. Without research, progress will stop. I see value in pursuing clinical trials immediately after you learn of your diagnosis, regardless of the severity of your condition. If doctors detect your cancer early, then you can join a clinical trial to complement your present treatment for better chances at remission or recovery. If your cancer is in its advanced stages, then there are two possibilities. Either your outlook improves because of the use of a new drug, or, while there is no benefit to your situation, your contribution will help future patients.

Find more information about clinical trials in the resources section R23.

CHAPTER FOUR

COMPLEMENTARY AND ALTERNATIVE MEDICINE

The National Center for Complementary and Alternative Medicine defines complementary and alternative medicine (CAM) as "a group of diverse medical and health-care systems, practices, and products that are not considered being part of conventional medicine."

They don't enjoy the same level of attention and respect as conventional medicine. Scientific evidence of certain CAM benefits, effectiveness, and safety exists, while for many other practices within CAM, the evidence is weak or inconclusive. Complementary medicine and alternative medicine are different therapeutic approaches; they differ in their implications and acceptance by standard medical science.

Complementary medicine uses disciplines such as yoga, meditation, and others to go *along* or *after* your treatment. Sometimes, doctors recommend the use of such therapies to reduce the side effects of the conventional treatments. Alternative therapies use an array of natural products, including botanical and nutritional products in the form of dietary and herbal supplements, as well as vitamins. Natural products, although maybe safe for many people, become unsafe when they interfere with cancer treatment that uses chemotherapeutic drugs. Their use in this manner can cause the medicine not to work in the body. Many people can experience adverse side effects because these products since they may interfere with a few anticancer drugs, making them not work as they should.

Complementary and alternative medicine (CAM) practices appeal to cancer patients through enhancing optimism and strengthening hope. The practices make them realize they have control over their cancer by playing an active role in their health. Unlike the choice limitations for conventional treatments, practitioners don't restrict a patient seeking CAM to specific therapies since they're always available and an accessible choice.

Research on CAM has not been adequate because of time, funding, regulatory issues, and the lack of finding institutions to work on the studies, making them harder to test due to the lack of scientific backing. Poor scientific support does not imply CAM therapies are not valid.

It's helpful for you to study and gather information about complementary and alternative medical practices related to your specific situation. Also note that certain therapies can be used for *both* alternative and complementary therapies, such as meditation or the use of some natural products. This research will help you make essential decisions on unconventional cancer treatment options. Use caution should you consider CAM practices alongside your present treatment, and especially if you wish to use them instead of conventional treatment. Consult with your oncologist before attempting to accept such methods. In the following few pages, I will cover these two practices in more detail. [R24]

COMPLEMENTARY MEDICINE

Complementary medicine is a useful adjunct to mainstream traditional medical care as a supportive measure to control symptoms. A few complementary approaches enhance well-being and contribute to the overall patient care by improving the outcomes of treatment.

It isn't a replacement for conventional cancer treatment, but it may lessen the side effects. Research studies performed on complementary cancer therapies found proof that a few health approaches may relieve cancer symptoms, but no evidence they can cure cancer. It's difficult to generalize the effects of using some complementary therapies on cancer patients when used alongside cancer treatment since people react differently to various treatment situations. If you have questions about alternative and complementary therapies, contact the National Center for Complementary and Integrative Health (nccih.nih.gov). The dedicated professionals at NCCIH would be glad to address your concerns and answer all your questions. Also, your oncologist should be one of the leading resources for your information.

The following list includes examples and brief descriptions of various complementary therapies that can be used alongside or after conventional cancer treatment.

Acupuncture uses many thin metal needles inserted into the skin at specific points on the body. Often, the practitioner applies electrical stimulations to the needles. CAM practitioners can use acupuncture to reduce nausea, vomiting, pain, and dry mouth after radiotherapy for head and neck cancers and ease the effect of hot flashes. Using electrical stimulation in acupuncture sometimes works, although its benefits were absent when studied in multiple trials. One way to avoid harm is by using clean needles.

Traditional Chinese medicine therapy uses a standard combination of herbs or botanicals used in many areas of Asia for a variety of illnesses. These products can reduce the toxicity associated with conventional anticancer therapy. As with acupuncture, no scientific proof backs their effectiveness. One herb used in this treatment is ginger to reduce and help control nausea because of chemotherapy. Sometimes, practitioners use it as a mix of anti-nausea medication.

Hypnotherapy is a safe way to make you forget your pain by altering your state of consciousness. It resembles daydreaming. You won't be asleep while you are undergoing hypnosis. You'll be in a state of heightened imagination. Scientific proof exists of its effectiveness in producing positive results in many patients who suffer from anxiety, pain, or nausea, through anecdotal patients account. Those patients confirmed that their cancer went into remission after the use of hypnotherapy. But remission does not mean cure. Again, there is no research data to establish that hypnotherapy can cure cancer.

Visual or guided imagery is a relaxation technique. The practitioner encourages the patient to relax by focusing on calming thoughts or experiences by imagining a friendly past event. This therapy was effective in women patients receiving chemotherapy for newly diagnosed breast cancer. When using relaxation training and guided imagery, these patients had a better quality of life when compared with a patient that used only chemotherapy.

Massage therapy may help to relieve symptoms of cancer such as pain, nausea, anxiety, and depression. It involves massaging parts of the body to relieve pressure. Research on massage therapy still lacks scientific proof. But whatever little information gathered suggests precautions are necessary when used as a cancer therapy. A massage therapist should consult with your doctor before performing massage therapy on you to learn to avoid pressure areas where the skin is sensitive because of treatment, especially for regions over the tumor.

Spirituality and religion can help religious or spiritual patients when grouped with conventional cancer treatments. Research showed that using religion and spirituality helps certain people in reducing the impact of some cancers' side effects, but only a few studies have showed its effectiveness (chapter 12). They can be useful for some patients. If you are not religious nor spiritual, then this therapy won't be helpful.

Yoga is a physical activity believed to lessen fatigue in some breast cancer patients. It has been documented to help with improving anxiety, stress, and depression. Yoga may produce unwanted outcomes in individuals because of its physical nature, so let your doctor know of any changes that may develop during therapy.

Meditation is a practice that resembles deep concentration when you focus on a special event. You may visualize a pleasant image, a sound, a place, or a cheerful idea. This technique relaxes your mind and body and trains your attention and awareness. The purpose is to achieve an emotionally calm state. It's used to relieve stress and anxiety. You can perform meditation alone or with other people.

Music therapy places you in a musical environment. You could listen to music or even play instruments if you know how to play. Your therapist will design your sessions to meet your specific needs. Meetings could be individualized, or they could be in group settings. You don't have to be a musician to be involved. It can help with nausea, vomiting, anxiety, and depression.

Tai Chi is an exercise that requires gentle movement of certain parts of the body in the form of light workout. It's a low-impact, slow-motion exercise that incorporates gentle movements and deep breathing. This gentle movement does not require exertion or strength, for example, breathing and focusing your attention on your bodily sensations. Your muscles will be relaxed, and connective tissues are not stretched during your sessions. People with disabilities and those who just had surgery can also do a relaxing technique to relieve many symptoms of cancer. Although Tai Chi is described as gentle movements of the body, it's recommended that you still consult with your oncologist before you perform such activity.

Relaxation techniques are methods to relax your mind and body. This treatment is used by concentrating your interest in calming your mind and unwinding your muscular tissues. These techniques may be comprised of tasks such as visualization exercises or modern muscle relaxation. Relaxation techniques might help relieve anxiety and also fatigue. They might likewise assist you to rest much better. Relaxation strategies are safe. A therapist leads you through these exercises, and at some point, you may have the ability to do them by yourself or with the help of guided relaxation recordings.

PLACEBO EFFECT

Placebo is a fake drug used alongside conventional treatment to find the outcomes of a study. It helps researchers understand the effect of a new medicine on a specific condition. Placebo isn't real medical treatment; it resembles a pill, shot, or other forms of treatment and does not contain active substances. Placebo can have positive and negative effects on the body, but the effects are not severe and can be controlled by doctors.

When the person has more symptoms or side effects after administering a placebo, it's called nocebo. It's a concept that involves a substance that sends messages through the nerves. When the patient is anxious or worried, the substance is activated, which triggers more pain than in a patient who isn't concerned. The concept of nocebo isn't fully understood, but research studies are ongoing.

Doctors use a placebo to understand the outcomes of certain situations when trying to test the advantages of interventions for cancer and related symptoms. Although these fake drugs don't act on the disease, the result of administering them to patients may have specific effects on how people feel, and it happens in one out of three people. These effects may generate or change the person's symptoms because of getting a placebo; hence, the placebo effect.

Researchers also use a placebo effect or placebo in clinical trials to compare standard treatment plus placebo, standard procedure plus a new one, and when the standard treatment is unavailable. Although a placebo isn't an active medication, they resemble the medicine under study. Using a placebo in this way can help patients and their doctors figure out their assigned treatment group.

Well-designed comparative research studies include a placebo treatment, besides an actual treatment to set up a distinct base between the two. For instance, a CAM therapy claiming to improve signs and symptoms of nausea or vomiting in half of the patients is of little help if placebo therapy improves signs and symptoms in half of the patients. They give a drug to specific patients to lower their cholesterol level, and others get a placebo as an example used to decide the effectiveness of the drug. Neither of the two groups knows if the treatment is fake or real. Researchers then will compare the results of both groups. That way, they can figure out the effectiveness of the drug and check their side effects.

Although the placebo effect is useful, it can create a problem when distinguishing its results from the results of the actual drug used for the treatment during a study. The distinction between the placebo effect and the effect of treatment may aid in improving the outcome and reduce the price of the drug testing. More research studies may lead to new methods to use the power of the placebo effect in treating disease. [R25]

Placebo can also be a procedure—for example, surgery's placebo effect. This topic does not apply to cancer surgery; hence, it's beyond this book. Contact the American Cancer Society or the American Council on Science and Health, ACSH, if you need information about surgery's placebo effect.

ALTERNATIVE MEDICINE

Practitioners promote alternative medicine (healing techniques and belief systems) therapies as a full or partial replacement for conventional cancer treatment; they laud their effectiveness by using a special diet to treat cancer instead of traditional drugs. Alternative medical systems include homeopathy, naturopathy, traditional Chinese medicine, and a few others. Medical doctors don't recognize alternative medical practices as standard or conventional therapeutic approaches. The rejection is problematic in oncology since a delayed or interrupted traditional cancer treatment may diminish the possibility of remission or a cure. [R24]

Alternative medical systems were created long before the standard medical practices. Examples of alternative medical systems developed in the Western world include homeopathic and naturopathic medicine. Examples of methods in non-Western cultures include traditional Chinese medicine and Ayurveda.

The alternative medicine field is made up of four categories:

o Mind-body practices are therapies to enhance the mind's capacity to affect bodily functions and symptoms. This category of alternative medicine may resemble complementary therapies mentioned above, but they become alternative therapies instead of complementary when they're used to replace treatment. Practitioners consider other methods including meditation, prayer, and mental healing that use creative outlets such as music, dance, or art.

o Biologically-based therapies are biological substances and products such as vitamins, supplements, herbs, and other natural products—for instance, the use of shark cartilage to treat cancer.

o Chiropractic, osteopathic manipulation, and massage therapies are part of manipulative and body-based methods in alternative therapies. They stem from the manipulation and movement of one or more components of the body. Energy therapies are examples of the exclusive use of the manipulative and body-based methods. These involve energy fields and bio-electromagnetic-based treatments.

o Dietary ACTs is a Gerson regimen based on a strict schedule for injecting fruits and vegetable juice. Gerson regimen, developed by Dr. Max. B. Gerson, is based on diet, supplementation such as minerals, enzymes, and other dietary factors, and detoxification, including enemas and other treatments. Gerson regimen also includes macrobiotic diets that are low fat, including vegetarian diets that include many complex carbohydrates, selected vegetables (SV) blended, boiled, and freeze-dried, and products that claim to have immune-stimulatory and anticancer properties. ACTs can also comprise a variety of herbal medicines (botanicals), including essiac, ginseng, green tea, Flor-Essence tea, and other supplements, including coenzyme Q10, hydrazine, melatonin, shiitake mushroom extract, and thymus extract.

SAFETY ISSUES

Conventional cancer treatments undergo a rigorous evaluation to figure out their safety and effectiveness. CAM is still less known to medical doctors, and research is still lacking and considered to be in its beginning stages. Insufficient CAM research causes the therapies to appear inferior and lacking, hence raising safety and validity issues.

You can buy herbal supplements and vitamins off the shelf in a grocery store or pharmacy. The FDA does not have to approve them so others can sell them to the public. They can be harmful when patients take them by themselves or with other substances. A few supplements may interact and interfere with cancer drugs, leading to undesirable outcomes. They can produce similar harmful effects when people consume them in high doses, including vitamin C while going through chemotherapy or radiation therapy. High doses of vitamin C can be unsafe even for healthy individuals.

The NCI states, "The results of taking vitamin and mineral supplements, including antioxidants, during cancer treatment, are uncertain." The NCI encourages cancer patients to speak to their health-care service providers before consuming any supplements.

A 2010 NCCIH-supported trial of a standard shark cartilage extract, taken beside chemotherapy and radiation treatment, showed no help in patients with advanced lung cancer; neither did a smaller-sized research study in patients with advanced breast or colorectal cancers.

A 2011 systematic review of a research study on laetrile discovered no proof of its effectiveness as a cancer therapy. Laetrile, also called vitamin B-17, can be poisonous if people take it by mouth since it has cyanide.

When we incorporate CAM practices with conventional medicine, the result is integrative medicine (IM), which treats the individual, including facets of lifestyle. It stresses the therapeutic connection between the practitioner and the individual, strengthened by proof, and uses proper treatments. Integrative medicine can help cancer patients manage symptoms to reduce the effect of treatment and provide them with a good quality of life by reducing anxiety and pain.

IF YOU ARE CONSIDERING CAM THERAPIES

Even after you investigate the sought-after CAM treatment, always gather information on the practitioner you intend to visit through checking their licenses with the local, state, and federal certification boards. Remember, even though a practitioner advertises their practices as natural, it does not mean natural will work for you. On the contrary, it might hurt your cancer case. Check with your insurance company on coverage of CAM if you don't intend to pay for it yourself, and don't spend your money until you know the treatment can be helpful to your health.

Never substitute standard medical treatment with alternative therapy. You are the ultimate decision-maker on the treatment you wish to undertake. Remember, a naturopath or a natural medicine doctor cannot inject you with any drugs nor prescribe medicine unless he or she is also a medical doctor.

A recent research study revealed women with breast cancer who refused or delayed surgery in favor of CAM were much more likely to have cancer development and to die of their condition than those who go through immediate surgery. Likewise, women who did not follow through with hormonal treatment, chemotherapy, or radiation as guided were a lot more likely to have cancer progress or die than those who underwent the recommended therapy.

IF YOU ARE FAVORING CAM THERAPIES

Some CAM therapies can be useful only because people respond to various treatments differently and because of the contrast in our biological structures and immunity.

There are reasons cancer patients favor CAM approaches. They believe conventional treatments are suitable since they're safe and effective and based on scientific research and clinical trials. But they also think traditional health care often leaves physicians and other health-care providers with not enough time to spend with them during their cancer journey due to their busy schedules. This dilemma may lead to inadequate attention to dedicate to other areas in which patients may seek support when facing a threat of cancer.

Many CAM practitioners can offer their time and focused communication on the patient's priorities. Some patients find CAM therapies appealing to their values and beliefs on health and life. CAM often provides a more holistic approach to a patient's life and family, including concentration on compassion and quality of life, and often hope for results more promising than those offered by standard treatments. Cancer patients want and need all that.

Another reason for favoring CAM therapies is that diagnosis and treatment of cancer are exhausting and demanding experiences. Cancer patients try these approaches because it's enticing to them since they feel as if they are taking control and decreasing uncomfortable symptoms and side effects of the standard treatment such as pain, fatigue, and nausea.

Information from 2012, the National Health Interview Survey (NHIS), showed that 33 percent of adults and 12 percent of children use complementary health techniques. And the most-used approaches are natural products and dietary supplements, apart from vitamins and minerals. One of these products is fish oil, a natural product used by adults and children. For body and mind techniques, adults and children resort to chiropractic care or osteopathic manipulation, yoga exercise, meditation/reflection, and massage therapy. The following key points are a summary of the costs involved in using CAM therapies in the United States:

o Out-of-pocket spending on these techniques for Americans age four years and older amounts to an estimated $30.2 billion, according to information obtained from the NHIS.

Expenditures are comprised of:

o $14.7 billion for visits to complementary and integrative health and wellness specialists
o $12.8 billion on natural products

o $2.7 billion on self-care approaches such as holistic medicine and self-help products

These out-of-pocket spending on complementary health approaches represent 9.2 percent of out-of-pocket expenditure by Americans on health care ($328.8 billion) and 1.1 percent of overall health-care costs ($2.82 trillion).

That is a huge chunk of money being spent on a field within the health care system that is not even endorsed by the medical community.

WHO PAYS FOR YOUR CAM THERAPIES?

A few insurance companies will only pay for proven methods of treatment, where others may pay for specific CAM therapies. Ask your oncologist for a letter of recommendation detailing the benefits you may gain from taking such measures for your cancer before you speak with your insurance agent. Your insurance company may consider such a letter and award you the insurance you need if it is convincing enough.

Some health insurance companies don't compensate you for using complementary health approaches, which may influence your decision to seek CAM. Researchers examined 2012 NHIS data on acupuncture, chiropractic care, and massage therapy, and compared it to data from 2002. While usage rates for the three approaches climbed, the increase among those who lacked having insurance was substantial. For those who had health insurance, coverage was more likely to be partial than full.

Some insurance companies might include insurance protection for complementary, alternative, and integrative practices if you ask them. You ought to find out if you need a particular rider or supplement to the standard plan for these approaches if you wish to include them in your coverage. You also should learn if the insurer offers a discount program in which plan participants pay for products and charges out-of-pocket, but at a reduced rate. Most likely, you may have to pay for CAM therapies yourself.

SO, IS CAM AN OPTION FOR YOU?

CAM approaches, or, more specifically, *complementary* procedures may be an option for you to consider anytime during or after your treatment to lessen the side effects. But they should never be a substitute for standard therapy.

The cancer journey is a managed process to ensure your safety. Doctors must learn of your interest in pursuing therapies outside conventional practices; they have legal and ethical obligations when discussing such avenues with the patient. Insufficient patient education and lack of communication during consultations between patients and doctors become obstacles, limiting any progress in a medical setting. It's then your responsibility to gain the knowledge to help in making informed decisions.

Your doctor may or may not choose to advise you against the use of alternative medicine for your situation. It's ultimately your choice to listen to your doctor. While most alternative and complementary therapies won't help your cancer, some might. Patients interested in pursuing CAM therapies should:

- Know the difference between alternative and complementary approaches.
- Establish excellent communication with the primary doctor, oncologist, and the rest of the health-care team members, including oncology physical therapists and nutritionists. The proper interface allows health professional to recommend the best complementary treatments for your case, if there are any. There always should be a balance between conventional medicine and alternative or complementary approaches, and your doctor is the best resource to establish such a balance.
- Study the benefits and risks of the therapy you choose. Specific treatments may have both risks and benefits where, in this case, you must weigh the benefits against the risks.
- Get a second, even a third opinion from different medical doctors who have prior training in the integrative field of medicine.

- Search a few qualified CAM practitioners with a successful history. Find out if they belong to a professional organization and whether they have a good reputation.
- Ignore CAM businesses that claim they can cure your cancer. Many complementary practices will help with the side effects of treatment, but they're not a cure for cancer.
- Talk to other people who may know about CAM therapies. Some of them may be educators or even individuals who have performed research on the subject or even patients who tried CAM therapies.

There are two kinds of medical doctors when discussing CAM, biased and non-biased. Biased doctors believe that patients should only abide by the conventional methods (surgery, chemo, and radiation) and ignore everything else unless clinical trials prove it and the FDA approves it. Non-biased doctors and the ones with education in integrative medicine will work with you and offer their sincere advice.

CHAPTER FIVE

SPECIALIZED CANCER CARE

Muhammad Ali once said, "Don't count the days, make the days count." These words are a perfect description of specialized cancer care in the form of palliative and hospice care. There is no reason your days as a cancer patient shouldn't incorporate happiness, joy, hope, and a good quality of life. Doctors have created unique types of care to provide you and your family with an experience to be as healthy as possible during the cancer journey. There are two main types of specialized cancer care:

- o Palliative care is designed by cancer professionals as noncurative treatment. It's to help you live as healthily as possible during all your survivorship phases, starting at diagnosis. Palliative care can be used alongside or after treatment to help ease the side effects you'll experience.
- o Hospice care is also a noncurative treatment, but it's only used in the months, weeks, or days before death. It aims at making your transition to the end-of-life period less uncomfortable for everyone involved, including your caregivers and family members.

These two types of care are not designed to cure your cancer or make you hope for remission. They are merely noncurative treatments made up of specialists from several disciplines; all work together to provide the needed care and add another layer of support. Palliative and hospice care services are useful for the patients, caregivers, and family members. The quality, professionalism, and expertise offered by the experts can also play an important role in reducing the stress patients experience during all phases of survivorship. The rest of this chapter explains these two types of unique, specialized care for all the parties involved.

PALLIATIVE CARE

This is a distinct support system, also called *supportive care, comfort care,* and *symptom management.* It improves the quality of life of patients having chronic illnesses, including cancer. It addresses the person, not just the disease, with emphasis on preventing or treating both symptoms of the disease and the impacts of its treatment. Palliative care also focuses on the physical, emotional, social, and spiritual issues cancer patients face during their cancer experience. Health-care personnel offers this care in a hospital, an outpatient clinic, a long-term care facility, or at home, always under the direct supervision of a physician.

Palliative care is comprised of a multidisciplinary team of specialists, including doctors, nurses, dietitians, pharmacists, chaplains, and psychologists. They all work in harmony with the primary oncologist and the oncology team overlooking your cancer situation to get the job done. Other members of the team include trained volunteers dedicated to providing caregiver support and facilitate communication among all the care team members.

When an individual gets palliative care, he or she may continue with cancer treatment, given they are both traditional medical approaches accepted by the medical community.

The care team is well-trained to provide patients with the best care through their understanding of the disease and the side effects of treatment. The team not only specializes in relieving symptoms of cancer, but also can help with other related issues, such as when you are feeling overwhelmed by complicated medical information, or the confusion or worry that may arise about making critical treatment choices.

Palliative care professionals have both the time and the knowledge to interpret the intricate medical details you get from your oncologist; they can help you understand what it all means—and what it all means for you.

The good news is that since the team specializes in managing a full range of signs and symptoms, they can make sure you enjoy the best quality of life possible. They'll help you figure out your immediate worries—such as stressing over how chemotherapy or radiation could make you feel, the impact of surgery, or what will happen if you end treatment. They will also help you with the bigger picture when deciding on what you value most in life or weighing the effects of therapy against those of the disease itself.

Palliative care is beneficial in the following cases:

- When you are seeking, receiving, or just completed treatment
- When you are managing cancer as a chronic (ongoing) illness
- When you have joined clinical trials to improve the outcomes
- When an occurrence is likely, when cancer is aggressive, or you are nearing the end of life

Research studies showed that integrating palliative care with the patient's usual cancer care may prolong survival and improve quality of life and mood. It also showed that this is possible if implemented after the diagnosis of advanced cancers. Research studies also proved that the use of palliative care could extend the patient's life by three months longer than patients who did not use it. The American Society of Clinical Oncology (ASCO) advises that all patients with advanced cancer receive palliative care.

Palliative care also addresses issues that may arise during your cancer experience. It discusses integrating your specific needs into care, taking into consideration your physical, emotional, spiritual, and practical needs.

Practical needs include financial and legal worries, insurance questions, and employment concerns. A palliative care specialist can talk to the caregivers regarding advance directives (R56) and help promote interaction among family members, caretakers, and members of the oncology care team to address these issues.

Palliative care is case-specific, and it changes over time while your situation is developing. If your oncologist diagnosed you with cancer or you just started therapy, palliative care can help relieve aggressive and adverse effects related to the treatment. It could reduce pain, nausea, and other physical symptoms. After cancer treatment, your palliative team will provide you with ongoing support to enhance the quality of life.

Research studies have confirmed that patients who had hospital-based palliative care visits spent much less time in a critical care unit. These findings showed that they were much less likely to be readmitted to the health-care facility after they went home. Studies also showed that individuals with chronic ailments like cancer who get palliative care have much less severe symptoms. They enjoy less discomfort, shortness of breath, depression, anxiety, and nausea or vomiting. Their health-care team often try to align with their values, goals, and objectives.

Specialists can aid caregivers, friends, and families deal with stressful situations to manage the circumstances and provide them with the help they require. Caregivers face many challenges, such as stress, especially if they're family members of the cancer patient. It's natural and typical for a family member to become overwhelmed by the extra responsibilities placed upon them if the patient faces physical impairment of any sort. Many caregivers and family members are confused about what to do, and they will need help in managing their own life while helping the patient. Addressing these issues is necessary so as not to compromise the caregiver's health, which may affect the patient's outcomes. [R26]

A specialized form of palliative care is called *palliative chemotherapy*, which can prolong the survival and ease symptoms of terminal cancer patients. Again, the purpose of palliative chemotherapy isn't to cure cancer. Oncologists recommend chemotherapy for two reasons—to get rid of cancer, which may not return (including some types of lymphomas and leukemias), or to control the size of the tumor after cancer has spread to other locations in the body, thus eliminating distressing symptoms caused by disease.

Before you decide on getting palliative chemotherapy, understand some terminology such as the *response rate* and the *median duration* of the proposed chemotherapy (see getpalliativecare.org)

The response rate is the potential that your cancer will improve from the treatment. If fifty patients were treated, and in twenty-five of them, tumors were reduced in size by half or more, then the response rate is 50 percent. Sometimes, the response rate can be expanded to include those patients whose cancer did not shrink, but also did not grow.

Median duration is the measure of how long your cancer is expected to respond to chemotherapy before cancer grows again. Patients with a more extended response are expected to live longer.

Before you decide on palliative chemotherapy, it's essential to understand the goals of treatment. You must have realistic expectations, make sure you are not thinking, or wishing, for results that aren't consistent with this treatment. Never seek a cure because of this treatment, even if your oncologist does not talk to you about the goals.

But if you go along with palliative chemotherapy, consider what the targets would be for you and understand that this treatment may or may not relieve symptoms. Sometimes palliative treatment can slow the progression of your cancer, hence extending your life. Overall, it can improve the quality of life because of reducing or eliminating some adverse effects caused by disease. Train yourself to ask your oncologist to explain the possibility of lengthening or shortening your survival, duration of the treatment, cost, time before seeing results, whether taking such a measure would disqualify you from joining clinical trials, and anything else that comes to mind.

HOSPICE CARE

Hospice care is the version of top quality, compassionate care that aids you and your family members in living as happily as possible during the end-of-life period. Any patient facing a life-limiting illness or injury can enjoy hospice care, not only cancer patients. It is comprised of team-oriented professionals and experts from various disciplines, along with the patient's medical care team members. They work together to tailor hospice care to the specific patient to provide all aspects of support needed to ensure a comfortable, pain-free quality of life. Everyone involved, including family members, loved ones, and caregivers receive support. It follows the philosophy that each one of us may die pain-free and with dignity.

Hospice isn't a building or medical facility. It's the care for cancer patients they receive at a hospital, in the home, a nursing home, an apartment, or any assisted-care facility.

People often confuse hospice care with palliative treatment. Hospice is for individuals with incurable diseases, used when therapy isn't working, and for those during the end-of-life period. Hospice care workers, although specializing in terminal cases, are also trained to provide palliative care during the disease, not only at the end of life. Medical health facilities offer hospice when therapy can no longer manage a health problem.

When you are close to the end of life—when you have less than six months to live—the aim is to comfort, not healing. Hospice care does not restrict patients to six months of services, as many believe. The following is what the National Hospice and Palliative Care Organization say about the time limitations:

- The Medicare Hospice Advantage requires that an ill individual has a prognosis of six months or fewer. There isn't a six-month limitation to hospice care treatments.
- Don't confuse hospice eligibility with the duration of the care.
- A patient in the final stage of life may receive hospice care, if required, when the doctor certifies that he or she continues to meet eligibility requirements.
- Under the Medicare Hospice Benefit, an endless number of sixty-day periods may follow two ninety-day durations of treatment, until the patient wishes to stop for whatever reason.

Some delays in pursuing hospice care come from patients and family members since they think hospice means the end of the road. The argument isn't correct. You can leave hospice and enter active cancer therapy should the need arises because of improvement with your situation. The hope is that hospice brings in quality life, making the finest of each day throughout the last stages of advanced illnesses.

Services provided by hospice care are like other supportive care, but with different approaches. Many care facilities keep essential staff members who have the training necessary to work in such an environment; hospice care staff members are accommodating and compassionate. Their work environment demands a certain quality that the specialist must have to gain the trust of the patient.

Hospice care members comprise an interdisciplinary health-care team to dictate the management. The unit may include a hospice doctor or medical director, and the care process may also include your family doctor. Other members are nurses, social workers, counselors, home health aides, clergy, therapists, and trained volunteers. The coordination between all members of your team is of high quality, done through a well-designed communication route.

Listening and helping patients, caregivers, and family members with various issues (for example, financial and emotional matters) are micromanaged with the highest accuracy. Volunteers play an essential function in the planning and offering of hospice care; they might be health-and-wellness specialists or ordinary individuals that assist in services ranging from hands-on care to help in the office or fundraising.

Coordination and information sharing among the care team members is essential. They must make sure that all involved services share information. The hospice team supervises and coordinates all services. These services may include the inpatient facility, the doctor, and other community professionals such as pharmacists, clergy, and funeral directors. The patient and caretakers are urged to contact the hospice team for issues of any sort, any time—twenty-four hours a day. Hospice care personnel assure you and your family you are not alone, and you can receive help. Some special services offered by the hospice care team are respite care and bereavement care.

Respite care is provided for caregivers, family members, or other individuals who are taking care of the cancer patient. It's intended to relieve them of some of the emotional burden imposed on them when caring for the patient, especially if the patient is a loved one. Caregivers might get burned out or show signs of stress and depression, where a break becomes necessary. It gives them time off to relax away from the environment of patient care.

There are two types of respite care; in-home care and residential care outside the home. In-home respite care means a family member or a friend assumes the responsibilities of taking care of the patient while the primary caregiver is away. Sometimes a professional can replace the primary caregiver for added convenience and quality or complex tasks. Other forms of respite care include nursing homes or hospices where the patient is taken care of by professionals until the primary caregiver returns. More specialized respite care exists for special situations, such as for serving disabled patients or for seniors.

Bereavement care is a service offered in the period of mourning after a loss. It's a service to help family members and caregivers in the grieving process. Other professionals may join the supervising hospice team from a different discipline such as trained clergy, volunteers, or professional psychologists to help with the situation, depending on the complexity of the issue. If your caregiver or family members require medical care, then the hospice team will refer the case to the specialized medical team to handle the situation. Bereavement services can continue for about a year after the patient's death.[R55]

As stated above, there are different locations where the patient can receive hospice care. Most patients prefer to get this care at their homes where they can enjoy the added convenience of having someone like a family member look after them. While this comfort is incredible, it can be a problem if the caregiver has a full-time job, children, other family members to care for, or any other responsibilities that may be an obstacle to constant monitoring. This problem can be solved through creative scheduling and teamwork among all those working to care for you.

A medical team of doctors, nurses, other specialists, and volunteers, still supervise home hospice care, no matter where your care location. While at home, the patient will receive visits from a specialist. Medicare-certified hospices must provide nursing, pharmacy, and doctor services around the clock. Some hospitals also offer hospital-based hospice that maintains a specialized hospice unit, or it could be a hospice team visiting patients with advanced disease in any nursing unit. Either way, the patient will enjoy the convenience of having the medical staff to offer their support around the clock to help control the symptoms.

Many nursing homes and other long-term health-care facilities keep small hospice units designed to host terminal patients. If they don't have the full capability or the required staffing to handle such a job, they might arrange with home health agencies or any other independent community-based hospices to provide the needed service to live-in patients. This option is excellent for individuals who don't have relatives or caregivers to care for them at home. Many communities and free-standing, independent businesses provide hospices that may be inpatient or outpatient facilities.

Before any hospice care facility admits the patient, he or she must sign a statement showing that the choice of a hospice care facility is their own. The doctor and the hospice facility medical director must also sign a statement attesting that the patient's remaining life is limited to six months or fewer if the disease runs its course. If the patient lives over six months while being cared for at the facility, he or she does not have to leave the program. They can continue being cared for if the medical director and the patient's oncologist approve extending care. Your health-care team will discuss your eligibility for attending a hospice care facility. They will answer your questions about insurance coverage and clinical trials while being cared for, and how insurance may affect your chances for hospice care or continuing services.

There is nothing trivial or straightforward about hospice care, but what patients must know is that hospice care isn't a surrender, nor is it about giving up. It's about living the remaining days, weeks, or months free of pain and improving the quality of life during those hard times

So, when is it a suitable time to join a hospice care program? When does the patient know it's the end? The answers are not simple nor straightforward, and the decision to join hospice care is personal. The patient should share it with family and close friends, and above all, he or she should inquire about it through the doctor and the health-care team. Ultimately, it's the patient's decision.

At a certain point in the cancer journey, when treatment stops working, the patient should rethink the situation. He or she must know another round of chemotherapy may extend life by another month, but they must consider that, during that month, the side effects of the treatment might cause more pain and agony. Sometimes, trying to enjoy the last few weeks or months of your life is an advantage you'll embrace over going through another round of chemotherapy. Note that even while you are in hospice care, you may still receive specific cancer treatments if your situation requires it. Hospice care will ensure that you are enjoying a good quality of life even while you are receiving treatment.

The American Academy of Hospice and Palliative Medicine has put together a list of signs that a patient may be ready for hospice care. These include:

- You've made several trips to the emergency room, and they stabilized your condition, but your illness continues to progress.
- The hospital admitted you several times within the last year with the same symptoms.
- You wish to remain at home, rather than spend time in the hospital.
- You are no longer receiving treatments to cure your disease.

Patients who fit these criteria can talk to their medical team to inquire about hospice care.

Who pays for hospice care services? Home hospice care costs are less than any other specialized facility like hospitals, nursing homes, or any institutions set up to provide such assistance. The low cost is because of the rising costs of technology and human resources needed to operate professional facilities. In a home setting, family and friends provide most of the help to the patients.

Many governmental and private institutions help with paying for hospice care, including Medicare, Medicaid, and HMOs. Donations from people in the community and gifts from non-profit organizations also help to provide free hospice care to cancer patients. There is always help available to everyone who needs hospice care. Some hospice facilities charge patients according to their ability to pay, and others may offer the service for free. [R27]

WHAT'S NEXT?

After diagnosis, your oncologist has told you whether your cancer is curative or noncurative.

If your cancer is curative:

- Go to chapter six, "Understand Your Diagnosis," and start gathering information about your specific cancer situation.
- Present the diagnosis data to another doctor and get his or her input. Find similarities and differences in both doctors' advice. If there are significant differences, then a third opinion is vital.
- Consult with past patients who had similar experiences, but remember that your situation is unique, so gain insight from those patients, but consult with your oncologist on your findings.
- Ask your doctor about your eligibility to join clinical trials and take advantage of palliative care, even at this early stage, to lessen the emotional impact of the diagnosis.
- Start improving your lifestyle habits (better nutrition, weight control, exercising, quit smoking if you are a smoker, stop drinking alcohol or drink in moderation) under the careful advice and supervision of your health-care team. Any positive change will be beneficial to your situation.

If your cancer is noncurative:

- Get a second and third opinion (if your financial situation allows it) and talk to other patients who shared similar experiences as yours.
- Depending on the results of all doctors' views, you may have to seek emotional and spiritual counseling.
- Ask your doctor about the possibility of joining clinical trials and investigate a few complementary therapies for further help to reduce side effects.
- Join a palliative care facility that meets your health requirements and financial status. Family and job factors may influence your choice when considering palliative care, but help is always available.

The long road ahead will be filled with obstacles, agony, and pain, but also pleasure and hope. Cancer does not mean a certain death anymore; it can be managed and maintained. Advances in technology and medicine are making cancer disappear slowly. There is an excellent possibility that you may become cancer-free and live a healthy life. Remember, cancer is a name used for over a hundred different diseases, and your case might be a simple form within the ensemble. Your cancer diagnosis is a landmark in your life; it begins your cancer survivorship journey. Best wishes.

> # PART TWO
> # THE STRATEGY

INTRODUCTION TO PART TWO

In part one, I provided you with basic cancer knowledge to help you understand your cancer situation.

The following chapters, 6–15, detail the strategy to help you self-manage your cancer journey, starting at diagnosis. Your position on the continuum determines your starting point. You can use the strategy at any stage of your cancer, regardless of its type. Consider yourself newly diagnosed if your cancer has resurfaced, or if you have developed a new primary cancer. In these cases, start at chapter 6, "Understand Your Diagnosis," again. Since you have prior experience in managing your disease, you may skip a few chapters and focus on the ones related to your new case.

Patients with advanced cancers where treatment does not work anymore, or where the body becomes resistant to cancer drugs, may wish to jump to chapter 15, "Restate Your Priorities," and never lose hope. In the rest of this introduction, I will outline all parts of the strategy in order. Each step of the strategy is explained in a full chapter and includes information about your current health situation and how to proceed from that point forward.

The name of the strategy is UNDOCANCER. Each letter designates the first letter of a step in the approach (something you must do). And each step constitutes a chapter in this book:

- **U**nderstand your Diagnosis
- **N**avigate your Treatment Options
- **D**iscover Available Resources
- **O**bserve your Health Needs
- **C**ategorize your Current Health in the Extended Phase
- **A**dapt to your New Health Needs
- **N**urture your Body, Mind, and Soul
- **C**ategorize your Current Health in the Permanent Phase

- **E**valuate your Life
- **R**estate your Priorities

The strategy is made up of nine steps, spread out in four main phases:

- Living with cancer (chapters 6, 7, 8, 9)
- Living through cancer (chapters 10, 11, 12)
- Living beyond cancer (chapters 13, 14)
- End-of-life (chapter 15)

Chapter 15, "Restate Your Priorities," does not apply to all cancer patients, only those nearing the end of life. I'm including this chapter as a part of the strategy since you are still considered a cancer survivor during the end-of-life period, although death can occur due to reasons unrelated to cancer. This chapter is beneficial for patients during the end-of-life duration, regardless of the causes of death or dying. After reading this summary, you can begin with the chapter specific to your cancer situation and continue from that point forward.

LIVING WITH CANCER

Living with cancer is also known as the *acute phase of survivorship*—when you have been diagnosed with cancer and are undergoing active treatment. This phase extends a few days after treatment is completed. Cancer treatment is the focus.

Chapter Six: Understand Your Diagnosis

Your oncologist just delivered the bad news about your cancer diagnosis. Although the word *cancer* is frightening, your specific diagnosis may not be as drastic as you think. Even if it's an aggressive form of cancer, the choices you make from this point forward will affect the outcomes.

Start with your oncologist and members of your primary healthcare team and ask a million questions. Go back to your original doctor, the one who referred you to the oncologist, and ask for a detailed explanation of the diagnosis. Get a second—even a third opinion, if your finances allow it. Despite all the answers, you'll still suffer emotional trauma that differs in intensity from other patients. Before you proceed any further into investigating your diagnosis, reduce the severity of the emotional shock and browse through part one of the book to learn the basics. After the psychological effects lessen, you must research your specific cancer case. This chapter shows you how to define your current position (diagnosis) within your cancer journey and what it means for your progress.

Chapter Seven: Navigate Treatment Options

Treatment relies on the type of cancer, stage, and other factors, including your age, current health condition, other diseases you may have, and so on. Sometimes, you can make choices concerning the treatment you wish to receive. You can even refuse treatment if that's your desire. But before refusing treatment, you must weigh the benefits and risks of halting treatment. Making the right decisions can substantially affect the outcomes, including your quality of life as a survivor. Study the side effects of each available treatment to minimize the negative impact on you and your loved ones. This chapter explains how to navigate your treatment options to make the most suitable one for your specific case.

Chapter Eight: Discover Resources

You cannot go through with your decisions on treatment and what to do afterward without proper guidance in the form of resources. Your most valuable resources are your oncologist and the assigned primary health-care team. But you cannot stop at that; your team members are serving many other patients and cannot dedicate their time only to your case. You must gain the skills to research further by using available resources to help you with your decisions.

You can find resources in abundance through well-known cancer organizations and academic medical institutions (listed in the resources section), along with books and medical journals. Your cancer may require not only health-care resources such as choosing the best oncologist and health-care facility, but also community support, social support, and spiritual resources. This chapter serves as a guide to give you a jump start with your search. Avoid resources claiming that they can cure your cancer.

Chapter Nine: Observe Your Health Needs

This period begins a few days after completing treatment. Here, you'll experience specific changes to your life that vary in intensity compared to other patients. Your emotional state is high, a lot is happening in your life, and you must observe emotional and physical changes after treatment and try to adjust. You may experience fear, anxiety, depression, and an array of other effects. Your physical changes will depend on the treatment or the mix of treatments you received. Surgery could produce varying results that differ in severity if changes to body parts were necessary for the best outcomes. Physical changes can add to your emotional trauma.

You must observe those changes and perform various activities (for example, changes to lifestyle habits) to maintain good health and minimize the possibility of recurrence. You are ready to leave the acute phase and transition into the extended period of your journey. This chapter focuses on psychological and physical changes after treatment and offers advice on how to lessen side effects by adapting to the new environment.

LIVING THROUGH CANCER

This is also known as the *transitional* or *extended phase* of the survivorship. It follows completing treatment. During this time, doctors monitor cancer for recurrence. The patient in this phase may also receive maintenance therapy. The effects of cancer and treatment are the focus. This phase is stressful for survivors.

Chapter Ten: Categorize Your Health in the Extended Phase

You have transitioned into the extended survivorship phase of the journey. The first follow-up visit's due now, where you'll learn about your progress and the results of treatment. Your oncologist has a good idea about your current health condition. Your situation can only fall under one of three main categories: cancer-free, in maintained remission, or living with the disease as a chronic illness. Each group has a set of health requirements and promotions. This chapter explains what your current health status means.

Chapter Eleven: Adapt to Your New Health Needs

The information here isn't reiterating chapter nine. Your psychological and physical conditions are changing, and you'll adjust to your health needs and become content with the changes after a few months after treatment. But you have temporary and permanent side effects that need dedicated personal attention, and some of them may require professional help.

Depending on your health condition, your oncologist will recommend the roadmap necessary for your initial wellness plan to help you with the future of your cancer. For some patients, some side effects may lessen or even disappear, and for others, they may stay for a long time. This chapter summarizes notable side effects and offers advice on how to either minimize or live with them.

Chapter Twelve: Nurture Your Mind, Body, and Soul

Your case-specific initial wellness plan details are not enough to cover the many aspects of your current and future health. You'll need more preparation to help you transition into the permanent survivorship phase, where you can continue self-managing your disease. This critical period demands added activities to strengthen your health promotions endeavor.

To execute health promotions, you must consider your body, mind, and soul as one and feed the unified entity with important events. Nurture yourself through becoming a volunteer, a cancer coach, or an advocate. Join community services and support groups to offer your experience to newcomers. This chapter shows you how to create or join such activities to feed your mind, body, and soul with the knowledge necessary to help yourself and others and to produce a better prognosis for yourself.

It's recommended that you engage yourself through becoming a cancer coach, a volunteer, an advocate, or by providing free cancer resources to others at *all phases* of your survivorship journey. These activities can educate you on your condition or on cancer basics that you can use to help others. But, primarily, the aim is to help you reach your hopeful goals for a better prognosis.

LIVING BEYOND CANCER

This period is when years have passed since cancer treatment ended. There is less of a chance that the cancer may come back. The focus of care is on the long-effects of cancer and treatment.

Chapter Thirteen: Categorize Your Current Health in the Permanent Phase

A few months have passed since you completed treatment, your health status is more stable now, and your oncologist will determine with some accuracy where you stand within your journey. This period is the watchful waiting time where you'll also be in fear of cancer coming back (recurrence) or having another tumor because of the treatment (chemotherapy, radiation therapy) you received.

You are entering the last survivorship phase to find out your new normal (and permanent) health category—you are cancer-free and asymptomatic, suffer from long-term or late-term effects, your cancer came back, or you have developed a second cancer. Each of the categories in this phase requires its specific set of health requirements and promotions. Your oncologist will offer you a case-specific wellness plan to ensure the best management of your condition.

This chapter explains the categories and the expectations of each. It also advises on specific health habits necessary to produce the best hopeful results from each health category.

Chapter Fourteen: Evaluate Your Life

You are doing your best and following your wellness care plan the best way possible, but you find that isn't enough. Fear, anxiety, depression, fatigue, and other psychological and physical conditions may remind you of your cancer every day, leading to possible distress. If you arrive at this point, it's an indication that your situation requires professional counseling and guidance. Doctors and psychologists cannot make a positive difference in your life unless you take charge of your health and open up about your true feelings.

You must now assess your life to find meaning in what's happening to you and your loved ones. To do that, you must discover and accept your *new normal* and make a few lifestyle adjustments to maintain the best health status in the new environment. It will be a long road ahead, strengthened by the valuable techniques of self-management that you have learned during the past few months.

Accepting what's happening to you through logical reasoning will only help you move forward. This chapter shows you how to search for your life meaning and give you the tools necessary to move forward and manage your disease as a chronic condition.

END-OF-LIFE

Chapter Fifteen: Restate Your Priorities

You have reached the end of the road. You may have stopped treatment for personal reasons, or your oncologist might have informed you that therapy isn't working anymore. It's time to restate your priorities to spare your family from heartache after your departure. During these difficult times, your emotional state may be at its highest, and your physical health may have deteriorated to a great degree. You need to lessen the severity of the emotional and physical trauma to ensure a peaceful transition into the end-of-life period.

This chapter guides you through preparing the legal documents you should complete as soon as possible. It also shows you other avenues to attain the best quality of life during the months, weeks, or even days before death occurs. During the end-of-life, the focus is on the quality instead of trying to prolong life.

The strategy outlined results from documenting actual experiences with my cancer patients. It's educational and practical. I have observed and studied individual reactions to the disease at various stages in patients who came from all walks of life. Some young lives were cut short and surrendered to this dreadful disease, while many others lived for many years after diagnosis. Some are cancer-free, and others are still self-managing their condition the best way they can.

Overall, I'm proud of the success achieved during my interactions with my patients. Education, embodied within passionate care and surveillance, is magical. Our beloved cancer patients are remarkable people who endured an agony that you can never visualize.

On the following page, I offer you a view from the top of the survivorship strategy, starting at discovery and running for the balance of life. It resembles the lifeline of your journey. You'll be able to find your position on the continuum according to your current health status and connect it to the chapter or chapters of concern. Note that the time indicated for each phase or category is only an approximation, and it may not be specific to your situation. Some patients may transition to the end-of-life period a few weeks or even days after treatment or even after diagnosis depending on the aggressiveness of their cancers. In these cases, the survivorship diagram does not apply, and other interventions are necessary.

You may find that multiple chapters share the same time interval (starting and ending times) or just the starting time during your survivorship phases—for example, chapters 10, 11, and 12. The similarity occurs because the same health promotions might be required at different places of your survivorship. Your health-care team members will be able to pinpoint the *exact* starting point.

Also, at the beginning of each chapter starting with chapter 6, "Understand Your Diagnosis," you'll see a diagram showing your starting point on the care continuum.

Introduction to Part Two // 81

U — Acute
- Understand Your Diagnosis - Chapter Six
- During your diagnosis meeting and shortly after

N — Acute
- Navigate Treatment Options - Chapter Seven
- Immediately after diagnosis until a day before treatment

D — Acute
- Discover Resources - Chapter Eight
- A few days after initial treatment is completed

O — Acute
- Observe Your Health Needs - Chapter Nine
- Starts a few days after treatment is completed

C — Extended
- Categorize Your Current Health - Chapter Ten
- Starts a few weeks after treatment is completed

A — Extended
- Adapt to Your New Health Needs - Chapter Eleven
- Starts a few weeks after completing treatment

N — Extended
- Nurture Your Mind, Body, and Soul - Chapter Twelve
- Starts a few weeks after completion of treatment

C — Permanent
- Categorize Your Current Health - Chapter Thirteen
- A year and more after completing treatment

E — Permanent
- Evaluate Your Life - Chapter Fourteen
- A year and more after completing treatment

R — Restate your Priorities – End-of-Life – Chapter Fifteen

THE ACUTE PHASE
LIVING WITH CANCER

CHAPTER SIX

UNDERSTAND YOUR DIAGNOSIS

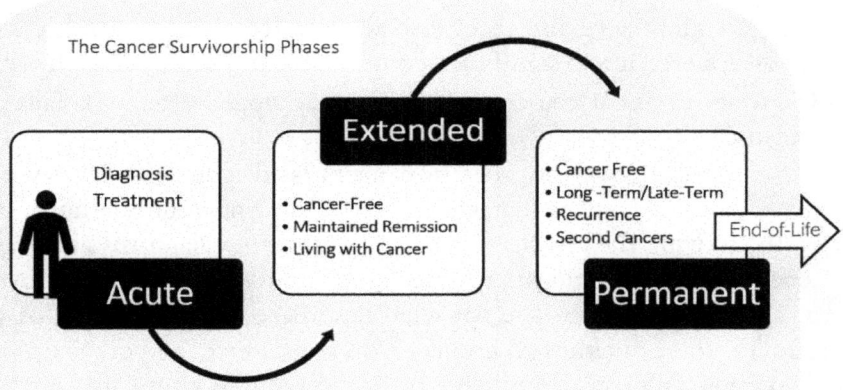

Your oncologist just explained your diagnosis

You are in the acute phase. Your oncologist just delivered the bad news about your cancer. You start asking questions and look for ways to ease your emotional trauma. This point is the beginning of your cancer journey; it's a critical time when you must understand the details of your diagnosis. Remember, your situation may not be as awful as you think

Many frightening diseases would kill you faster than cancer, but this beast is the most feared. A cancer diagnosis has a significant effect on you and your family members' health and well-being—your life changes in every sense, including your outlook on life. Your altered state of consciousness can produce devastating outcomes, should your condition lack proper professional guidance.

You may be harmed emotionally and physically upon receiving the news. It might be a deep ache in your chest, or it could be a profound feeling of emptiness, and you may feel instant isolation. No matter how you describe your emotions, it's challenging. The impact and the severity of hearing such disturbing news has varying degrees of effect on people, sometimes ferocious.

We all receive and react to bad news from our perspectives. It's all deciphered into a significant emotional—and sometimes physical—paralysis in most patients. It triggers a ripple effect of fallacious reasoning.

Knowledge of your specific cancer case diagnosis is the power you need to enable you to live with cancer. Knowing your condition starts with studying the results of your medical tests. Diagnosis and staging occupy the first phase of the cancer survivorship and must be examined to prepare you for what lies ahead. Upon learning of your cancer, you can either go home, sit on your couch, and cry like a baby, assuming failure is imminent, or do something about it—and do it now.

This chapter will take you through the moment of diagnosis, starting at your doctor's visit and going until you leave his or her office and a little beyond. It covers the period beginning with your diagnosis, and includes the next few days before you start your treatment.

Understanding your diagnosis isn't only limited to learning the medical terminology in your pathology report. It prepares you for the subsequent phases of your journey, including making treatment choices most proper for your health situation. There are still other vital elements to consider during this critical period. You must implement those factors during the few days after diagnosis while preparing to discover the most appropriate treatment options. They are:

- o Manage your emotional reactions after hearing the news about your cancer. The psychological shock can prohibit

clear and positive thinking if it isn't dealt with properly. Sometimes, professional counseling by a therapist may be necessary.
- Attend multiple meetings with your oncologist to learn the details of your report and outcomes of your situation.
- Gather more resources about your specific illness besides the information supplied by your oncologist.

THE EMOTIONAL SHOCK

Mental anguish and confusion because of having cancer will accompany you throughout your cancer journey, with variations in intensity, severity, and type. Responses to lousy news differ for different individuals. The following exciting and unusual story about a friend of mine, whom I have accompanied to his diagnosis meeting, will astonish you. It's puzzling to me.

My friend Mark was thirty-three years old at the time of his diagnosis, married, and a father of three small children. He was enjoying good health before receiving the news of his cancer. One morning, Mike woke up with a persistent stomachache that wouldn't go away, even after consuming several off-the-shelf medications.

Days later, after performing a few medical tests, he was referred to an oncologist, who then called him into his office to tell him he suffered from cholangiocarcinoma (bile duct cancer). His cancer was stage IV and very aggressive.

Mark asked me to accompany him to meet with his oncologist to help him understand the situation. After receiving the news of the diagnosis, I looked at Mark's face to examine his initial reaction. His response was more baffling to me than the actual diagnosis.

After he heard the news, he looked straight at me, not at his doctor, and said, "That sounds terrible, right, Sam?"

I started experiencing a shock of my own as a response to Mark's reaction, but I knew that I had to answer his question. I always have been truthful with my patients, taking into consideration their state of mind at the demoralizing moment. I confirmed his thoughts and responded with a yes.

"Oh, well. This is life. All we can do is try our best." He uttered his words with facial expressions that did not show excessive worry. "I guess this will change everything," he added.

The trip back to his residence lasted thirty minutes, during which there was nothing unusual about our conversations. He asked me a few questions about his diagnosis and inquired about a plan. His smiles and loud laughs were breaking the few quiet moments we had, a sign of what appeared to be a slight worry.

Despite Mike's reaction to the news, most common resentments include a multitude of psychological and medical conditions ranging from a simple upset and sadness to a more substantial response of crying, and even, in rare cases, fainting. Similar effects can be a challenge to loved ones. They may be worried about losing you and concerned about how they will be affected. Having people in your life who will suffer from emotional issues because of your cancer adds to your list of worries and traumatized emotions.

You'll discover that many people around you try to take the role of a doctor or a psychologist and educate you on your illness. Some people will say offensive words. They may be concerned about you but lack the skill to show their concern, resulting in unnecessary chatter. The bottom line is never listen to any advice unless it's coming from a professional.

Some others, even friends, may abstain from your company because of personal reasons and understandings. They might presume that being around you reflects what happens to them should they get cancer, and they want to spare themselves from such traumatic moments. Or, they may be afraid that showing their feelings may add to your list of worries. No one is to blame due to the chilling aspects of the situation, regardless of their reasons for not being present.

It may take a while to repair yourself and go back to reality, but it's essential to pave the way to infiltrate the next crucial few days of your journey, the treatment period. So how do you reduce the adverse effects as a response to your diagnosis?

Your body reacts to stress in a variety of ways. It's excellent if it's temporary, but if it lasts for an extended period, your body will respond to physical, psychological, or mental pressure by discharging stress hormones that raise blood pressure, speed heart rate, and elevate blood sugar levels. These responses are great since they help a person act with greater strength and speed to escape perceived threats. However, experiencing severe long-term (chronic) stress can produce digestive complications, fertility issues, urinary problems, and a weakened immune system. Individuals suffering from chronic stress are also more prone to viral infections such as the flu or common cold. They may also experience headaches, sleep troubles, depression, and anxiety.

Links between psychological stress and cancer could appear in several ways. People under stress may develop certain habits, such as overeating, consuming more alcohol, or smoking. They all increase a person's risk for cancer. If an individual has somebody like a family member with cancer, they might have a higher possibility because of a shared inherited risk factor—not because of the stress caused by the family member's diagnosis.

Those who attempt to regulate the problem with risky behaviors such as smoking, drinking alcohol, or becoming more inactive may have a more mediocre quality of life after cancer treatment. In comparison, individuals who can use effective coping strategies to deal with stress, such as relaxation and stress monitoring strategies, have been revealed to have reduced levels of depression, stress, anxiety, and symptoms associated with cancer and its treatment. There is no proof that effective management of emotional stress enhances cancer survival. Although there is still no reliable evidence, it directly affects cancer outcomes; some data suggest that patients can feel vulnerable when the situation becomes overpowering. But evidence from experimental studies shows that psychological stress can affect a tumor's ability to grow and spread.

This reaction is linked to higher rates of death, even though the mechanism for this outcome is vague. Maybe people who experience sad or helpless feelings don't pursue treatment when they become unwell. They may give up too soon or fail to adhere to likely reliable therapy. Also, they may engage in risky behaviors like drug use or refusal to preserve a healthy lifestyle, leading to an early death.

Stress becomes dangerous when it transforms into distress. Distress emerges because of mismanaging your emotional state. It's when you feel that you cannot control changes caused by cancer or handle normal life activities. It can reduce the quality of life. There is even scientific evidence that more unsatisfactory clinical outcomes can lead to extreme distress. If you feel that you are in trouble, then immediate medical attention is needed. Having these feelings can serve as an obstacle to managing your cancer.

Coping with psychological stress requires professional intervention. Support can reduce levels of depression, anxiety, and disease-and-treatment-related symptoms among patients. Various types of approaches have been adopted by doctors to aid patients in their psychological journeys, including relaxation and meditation techniques or stress management. Also, the patient could take advantage of cancer education sessions, social support in group settings, medications for depression or anxiety, and exercise.

Different types of counseling are necessary for various phases of the cancer journey, such as the pre-treatment and after-treatment periods, or at any point in the survivorship stage, including end-of-life preparation. Patients who show moderate-to-severe distress should consider relevant resources, such as a clinical health psychologist, social worker, chaplain, or psychiatrist.

It always helps to have a clear mind during this period of your cancer journey. You cannot ignore your emotional feelings at this phase, so take a break, revisit your state of mind, and repair any damages the news may have triggered. If you are in denial, then snap out of it. If you are incapable of relieving yourself from the anxiety or stress or any other symptoms, seek professional support before you study your cancer diagnosis. It will help if you aren't distracted. You'll need all your brain power to help you comprehend your cancer and be able to make alarmed decisions for the duration of the acute phase before making treatment choices.

Having cancer now makes you unique in every sense, and you have a ton of people to help you deal with it. The more cancer knowledge you possess, the more comfortable you'll be with your diagnosis. The more specifics you know about your cancer, the more relaxed you'll be. Combining knowledge and relaxation will give you the peace of mind you need to fight your disease. [R29]

HOW TO MANAGE THE SHOCK

Dealing with emotions may be difficult at first. After a cancer diagnosis, it can be a challenge to identify and honor your feelings. There is plenty you can do to gain control of the situation and eliminate stress. The good news is that you can do a lot on your own to reduce the severity of negative emotions. The following three steps are crucial to the recovery process. Start by accepting the situation, recognizing the problem, and finding emotional support.

Accepting your feelings: Acceptance is always the first step to solving any personal issue despite the magnitude or intensity of the situation. Denial increases the pressure on you, forbidding you from clear thinking. Accepting your cancer widens your horizon and allows you to take the next immediate step to think of a solution.

You can abstain from judging your feelings through spending time with interesting people who have a humorous nature to help you forget about your cancer, those who are positive and uplifting. Also, avoid being alone. Even if this is your nature, you must try to break the habit and be around people. Remember that many emotional challenges are temporary and will lessen or go away as you travel the continuum. Most negativity will diminish with time; your sense of hope and confidence will increase with each passing day.

Accepting your feelings will protect you against feeling lost and losing hope. Having a support system is a beneficial part of dealing with emotions. Your primary care team will always be your first line of defense against all your debilitating emotions.

A fundamental requirement for accepting your feelings is to embrace reality and understand that cancer affects millions, so you are not alone. These words may not be comforting enough, but knowing that you are not alone in this ordeal may help. You have cancer now, and you are a new person. Do what it takes to create an environment of acceptance.

Recognizing depression: Knowing your feelings is the second major step in pursuing relief from the shock. The National Institute of Mental Health defines depression as a "serious but common illness." Depression incorporates feeling down or hopeless for weeks at a time. You are at a heightened state of depression because of your diagnosis. Signs of depression vary for different people, but you could suffer from symptoms like feeling confused, overwhelmed even with the smallest things, have memory problems, issues with sleeping, fatigue, loss of appetite, and feeling sad and helpless.

Monitoring your depression will allow your health provider to test the extent of its severity and its effect on you. There are many ways your doctor can treat depression. Sometimes your doctor may change your depression medication to suit your situation. Other times, he or she may recommend more intensive and specialized counseling or both.

Many cancer patients blame themselves for having cancer. They think if they had made specific lifestyle adjustments, they would have avoided the disease. It's too late for the blame game. For the significant part, you did not cause the disease. You have cancer because something has created it. Perhaps you were part of the cause through your lifestyle, but maybe not. It does not matter now. You must deal with the problem. These thoughts can elevate your depression. Avoidance of such negative thinking will reduce your depression level.

Finding emotional support: Specialized support exists for your situation. Sometimes finding the most suitable support system can be tricky. Always investigate and ask your oncologist about your next step in finding the right support for you. Not all support systems and organizations are qualified to help you with your situation. The wrong support can only waste your precious time. Support systems and support groups can provide a safe place to share experiences with others who are dealing with cancer. If you have reached a point of determining that you need emotional support, this means you have recognized that you suffer from psychological trauma. And that means you have become a significant problem solver in your situation. The solution starts with you as soon as you acknowledge that you are suffering from emotional trauma. It's a great start.

Other practices you can perform that may have a meaningful impact on the outcomes include:

- o Organize your life and take it easy. You may have to change the course of your regular routines and start performing fewer activities so you don't exhaust your body. And don't mix activities. Mixing or combining activities requires more energy, causing unnecessary mental and physical exertion on your body.
- o Focus on essential tasks. Don't waste your time thinking about issues that are not related to your improvement. Overthinking can also be exhausting, so don't overwhelm yourself.
- o Prioritize your tasks and concentrate on the things that you can control. Avoid anything that causes stress, and take care of little and big ideas. You may need to dig into your financial situation and ensure that you are stable, perhaps through

contacting your insurance company or finding financial advice related to your case. If you cannot cover your bills because of obstacles, seek financial help from various specialized institutions. Your social worker can help you in this matter. Family, friends, coworkers, and associates are always there to offer their help in those difficult times.

- Minimize the number of stress factors in your life. By diminishing most stressors, you may not prevent stress, but these management techniques can help you feel more relaxed and less distressed. Spend time outside either by yourself or with someone close to you, such as a family member or your spouse. Attend social activities and offer your contribution within comfortable limits. Start a nutritional plan with the aid of your nutritionist or members of your health-care team. Sleep well, perform activities that relax your body and mind, and focus on a hobby and try to become good at it. Write, swim, travel, do whatever to keep you away from thinking about your disease.
- Relaxation by far is the best avenue to reducing your emotional trauma and clearing your mind. If you are incapable of relaxing on your own, then try to attend a few relaxation-technique sessions. Some relaxation techniques like deep breathing, mental imagery or visualization, progressive muscle relaxation, meditation, biofeedback, and yoga can help make you relaxed. Before you attempt to take advantage of these activities, consult with your doctor, especially when the technique you are pursuing is physical, as in massage therapy.

You can find more information on how to manage the emotional shock of diagnosis in the resources section R29.

YOUR DIAGNOSIS REPORT

Understanding your pathology report is a matter of utmost importance, but it comes with many obstacles when you try to make sense of the medical terminology that makes it up. When it's ready to be viewed by your oncologist, request that the report is available to you in a language you can comprehend. Medical words and terms such as *biopsy*, *grade*, *mitotic rate*, *tumor margin*, and others can confuse you and can distract you from learning your diagnosis.[R30]

Your oncologist will try to explain the wording of the report. Don't just listen to his or her explanations; ask questions about anything that might seem vague. Some doctors are not trained to communicate with patients and are not capable of translating the language of the report into layman's terms. If you find yourself trapped in this situation, seek further help from your health-care team members or talk to the experts at cancer organizations listed in the resources section under "General Cancer Resources."

Getting answers to your questions will give you a clear picture of the whole situation. Don't be shy or think your inquiry is irrelevant or stupid; every question or concern you may have is legitimate. Your doctor does not mind, and he or she will help address all your concerns. If you don't understand an answer to a question, ask him or her to explain the answer in a different method.

So, what kind of information does the pathology report contain? A pathology report includes data from examining cells or tissue under the microscope. Data collected from the sample examination enable the pathologist to find out if cells are noncancerous or cancerous. The pathologist can also find specific details about the tumor's features such as growth, shape, and appearance of a sample as it looks to the naked eye. This information is called *gross description*. It plays a vital role in cancer diagnosis and staging.

Completing the report may take several weeks before it's ready. Your doctor will receive the test results when they become available.

The anatomy of the report is comprised of seven main areas:

- o The general information area. It begins with an overview of your personal information such as your name, birth date, a personal identification number to identify samples, information about your doctor, and information on the sample testing laboratory. It also includes details about the specimen examined, such as the biopsy, surgery, or the tissue under consideration.
- o The second part of the report interprets the tissue sample of the tumor as seen by the naked eye. The name of this sample is *gross* or *obvious description*.

- The third part is the most scientific, called the *microscopic description*. It shows what the cancer cells look like when seen under the microscopic lens. This section includes the most valuable data affecting diagnosis and treatment. It includes details about your cancer size, shape, grade, how quickly cells are dividing (mitotic rate), tumor margin, stage of cancer, and whether it has spread to nearby lymph nodes or organs. This section may also contain information from other tests such as identifying specific genes, proteins, and may include additional information unique to the tumor under study.
- The fourth part of the report is the diagnosis information. It provides the bottom-line details. It includes information about cancer, lymph-node status, margin status, more information about the stage, and other results, such as whether the tumor has hormone receptors or other tumor markers.
- The fifth part of the report is the synoptic summary. The pathologist will include a review when he removes the entire tumor that specifies the most relevant results in a chart. These are the items taken into account that are most important in identifying a person's treatment alternatives and chances of improvement.
- The sixth part is the remarks section. Often, cancer may be difficult to detect, or the growth of the tumor is ambiguous. In these scenarios, the pathologist may use a comments section. Here, the pathologist can explain the issues and may recommend other tests. This section may also include additional information that can help the doctor plan treatment.
- The seventh part is comprised of the sampling variations. The pathology report for a biopsy may differ from subsequent findings for the whole tumor. This difference happens because the features of the disease can sometimes vary in different areas. Your doctor will consider all the collected data to aid in developing a treatment plan specific to you. The information in this part of the report further helps your doctor customize a specific treatment plan for your case.

Even after reading and studying your report, there will be a possibility that you don't understand everything listed in it. To help you clear the matter, ask questions about your cancer and its origination, how large is it, how fast it's growing, if it's invasive or noninvasive, whether it can be removed, stage, progression, prognosis, remission, and whether there's a chance of full recovery. [R30]

GET MORE INFO

Why should you try to gather more information about your illness? Isn't the information your doctor gave you through the diagnosis report and the many meeting you had with him enough? I mentioned earlier that some doctors may not be good communicators and are incapable of delivering the information in a format assimilated by nonmedical persons. Also, your doctor may treat other patients' cases with yours, so his total devotion cannot be only to your cancer case. Despite what your doctor tells you, and even though he may be the best doctor in town, you must seek more information about your case through the many available channels.

While there are many methods you can implement to gather case-specific information, such as bestselling books, medical journals, and the internet, always verify it with one of the well-known and trusted cancer organizations. Some trusted sources are: The National Coalition of Cancer Survivorship, (NCCS) [R1], The National Cancer Institute (NCI) [R2], the American Cancer Society (ACS) [R3], and the National Comprehensive Cancer Network (NCCN), as well as many other renowned cancer organizations worldwide, found under "General Cancer Resources."

These organizations and many others possess the qualifications and the trained personnel to steer you in the right direction. Internet websites claiming that they have a cure for your cancer have been created for commercial goals. Avoid them altogether.

Each phase of your survivorship and each step requires its unique information-gathering process, like information about treatment options, a wellness plan particular to your case, or self-management of your cancer as a chronic illness. The process can overwhelm, and it becomes involved whenever you must get information about multiple symptoms that you may experience at a later phase in the survivorship stage. Some data may include getting details about recurring cancers or second cancers in the permanent and chronic periods of your illness.

In this book, I will guide you through the information-gathering process for your current position on the continuum (where you are in your cancer journey) and offer convenient and straightforward techniques to gather such information. You must learn, in detail, your cancer—whether it's localized (benign) or malignant (can spread in the body), its origination and risk factors, and its causes. You may not get answers to all your questions now, but as time progresses, your oncologist will provide you with more insight when the results of the treatment are more prominent.

Take a few days. Rid yourself of the negativity that accompanies your emotional state of mind. Relax and concentrate on preparing yourself for navigating your treatment choices. Remember that asking specific questions about your cancer must be directed at the individuals who are most familiar with your situation, including your oncologist, your oncology nurses, and maybe other members of your primary health-care team. Professionals at cancer organizations can only answer general questions and offer recommendations for doctors at various facilities, but they cannot answer specific questions about your case.

The next chapter, "Navigate Your Treatment Options," prepares you to decide on the most suitable treatment for your cancer case.

CHAPTER SEVEN

NAVIGATE TREATMENT OPTIONS

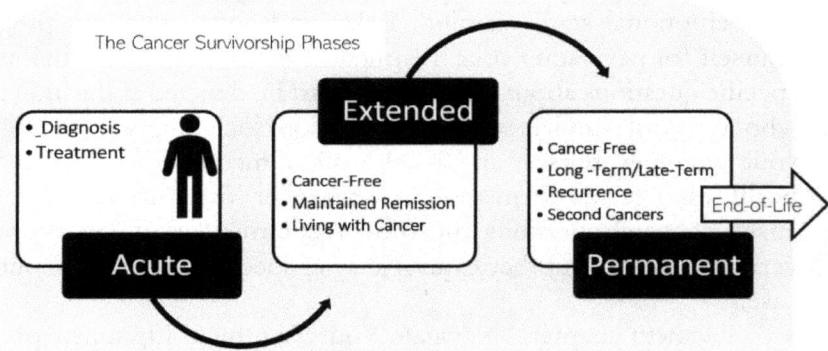

Now you'll choose the treatment(s) for your cancer

You are in the acute phase. It has been a few days since you received the news of your cancer diagnosis. You are trying to learn about the best treatment or a mix of treatments for your cancer. Choosing a treatment is your decision; otherwise, trust your oncologist. It's still recommended that you seek a second opinion even after you or your oncologist decide.

Are you ready to govern the focal point of your journey? The news about your cancer diagnosis has left you with emotional scars and kept your mind reeling. You have worked hard to clear the path for making important decisions about your treatment options. Your choices (if you have any) concerning treatment will impact the outcomes of your disease.

Deciding on treatment options may require you to involve a close friend or a loved one to engage in the decision-making process. Having a person to talk to and share information will lessen your burden and offer encouragement during this challenging time.

Should you learn about your prognosis before you decide on treatment options? What information do you need to help you reach the point of planning? What are your goals and expectations from such treatment? Reading this chapter, you'll have answers to all these questions.

Take a day to absorb the information and the results of your discovery process, then come back to start your treatment. Remember that it's your decision, should you favor no treatment or halt it at any point. But before you attempt to refuse or end treatment, please read this chapter to learn about the many dangerous consequences resulting from such action.

EXPECTED CHALLENGES

Cancer, being a complex system of single complex diseases, is one of the most significant challenges facing both the medical community and the patient. This challenge is more explicit in patients trying to decide on the best treatment options that are most suitable for their types of cancers—facing the many difficulties involves understanding the diagnosis and weighing the benefits and risks of treatment, as well as how the side effects will influence your daily life.

Going into treatment isn't merely signing the consent form to allow your doctor to start the process. You must do your homework to know what you are signing. You are ready to receive chemotherapy, radiation therapy, or both. Do you know the implications of such processes? Have you explored complementary therapies to go along with your treatment? Did you ask your doctor about the possibility of joining a clinical trial? Are your chosen physician and health-care facility the best for your specific situation and do they have experience treating conditions similar to yours?

Doctors come from all walks of life. Some of them are famous and experienced, and some others are neither known nor have enough experience to treat your case. Others have specific expertise in your cancer, and some others are just starting. Although they're all called doctors, some of them graduated top of their graduating class while others graduated last.

Does your doctor try to establish a distinct communication channel with you? Do they explain the situation well and have the time to spend with you to define the medical terminology in a form easily comprehended by you? How about giving you enough time to ask questions? Excellent communication can serve as a transparent window to producing better outcomes by enabling you to make informed decisions, making information flow simple. The same is true for your choice of the health-care facility where you'll receive your treatment. Investigating these choices can mean the difference between life and death.

How do you educate yourself on this complex subject? The complexity of the matter is substantial, so how can the layman assimilate the information that he or she must collect to help decide on the best treatment options? On the bright side, you don't have to go to medical school to comprehend such information related to your cancer case. Many health-care professionals and dedicated medical institutions have worked hard at simplifying the medical narrative into a form to be understood by the layman. Asking a million questions and continuing research will provide you with satisfactory answers to help you make informed decisions. Ask any question that comes to mind and know that your doctor does not mind your questions.

What are your preferences? Do you wish for an excellent quality of life through avoiding specific side effects, or do you prefer to prolong your life under any circumstances, even if this means enduring a harsh treatment? Often, this confusion can be a cause of conflict between doctors and their patients.

Sometimes, individual patients have reservations about the results of treatments like chemotherapy—for example, losing their hair (even if it's temporary), or a specific disfigurement to a part of the body (although it might not be visible to the public). You must discuss such quality-of-life issues with your doctor and ensure that he or she explains the consequences, should you be the one making all the decisions concerning treatment.

Other forms of challenges may arise during these uncertain times, including covering the cost of cancer treatment and whether your insurance coverage suffices. And job-related issues can surface, such as missing work, making things difficult if your job is your only source of income. Transportation could be an issue if you must travel long distances to receive treatment. You may face family problems if your new situation has resulted in imposing a burden on some family members. Challenges differ for patients; they vary in their intensity depending on the patient's physical, financial, and mental capabilities.

TREATMENT OPTIONS

Possessing the proper knowledge about your diagnosis and stage of your cancer allows you to define what you can expect from treatment. Your cancer type, location, and staging will restrict the specific kinds of treatments. Here, you have two options—either you go ahead with your doctor's recommendation or refuse it. Declining treatment is your decision, and no one can force you to do it if you choose not to endure the experience.

Now you have a general idea about what treatment choices are available for your specific case. You must understand which one (or a mix) is most suitable and if you have multiple options. Collect more information about each option and choose the one with fewer side effects. While there are a dozen different treatments in existence, the most popular methods are surgery, chemotherapy, and radiation therapy. Depending on your situation, you may be likely to receive a mix of two or even more for the hope of increasing the likelihood of getting rid of most of the cancer cells.

Cancer treatments have pros and cons. Inquire about this matter if the most appropriate choice for you is a surgery where disfigurement can be substantial or visible to others. Below, I summarize the leading cancer treatments. For more detailed information, refer to chapter 2, "Cancer Fundamentals."

Surgery: It may be the most viable option, depending on your specific condition, and it's the most popular method out of the three main, standard approaches. Surgical treatment is suitable if the tumor is large and simple to remove, depending on your cancer, its stage, and location in the body. If cancer has metastasized to other parts of the body, then surgery isn't the best option, and it may not even be an option. Healing from surgery (large incisions) may take a long time, accompanied by infection and excessive bleeding for some patients.

Chemotherapy: This practice uses drugs that destroy cancer cells. Doctors administer this procedure by injecting the body with drugs that suppress cancer cells. It works by keeping the cancer cells from growing, dividing, and making more cells. It slows down the growth of the tumor. The problem with chemotherapy is that it also kills healthy, living cells in its path, which causes some unwanted side effects.

Radiation therapy: Killing cancer cells through radiation is another method to treat cancer. Doctors can administer it from outside the body (extra beam radiation) or from within (brachytherapy). It isn't a reliable option for all kinds of cancers, but it's ideal for a single tumor or mass. With radiation, immediate side effects are likely to be less extreme than those of chemotherapy.

Not everybody profits from the most known forms of cancer treatments. For several types of cancer, some other, less frequently used approaches may be more efficient. Some of those treatment options include biological therapy, hormone therapy, targeted therapy, immunotherapy, and photodynamic therapy.[R31]

DECISION TIME

When you consider all treatment options available for your specific cancer with your health-care team and loved ones, you must determine what you can expect from treatment. Deciding about the most suitable treatment isn't arbitrary. There are guidelines you should consider while making the most alarming choices, including:

Setting up your ground rules: Like anything else in life, you must establish rules and adopt strict regulations unique to your situation. Success may not be attainable without guidelines that you must follow. You set ground rules after you learn about all your treatment options. Familiarize yourself with various types of treatments to enable you to make an uncomplicated final decision.

How much do you want to know? Would gaining more information make you uncomfortable and hesitant? Understanding the statistics and survival rate for your cancer may not be okay for you. Some patients can make decisions that most suit their needs if they know more, but some others are the exact opposite. Decide whether pursuing such action about future outcomes would be helpful or unfavorable considering your emotional state at the time of the inquiry.

Do you know someone else, such as a family member, a close friend, or even someone else who knows about various cancer treatments who can accompany you while you talk to your doctor about your options? Some people will gain more confidence in knowing there is somebody they can confide in attending with them during the decision phase. If you feel that you need someone to be there with, tell your doctor.

Do you want to decide? Or would you prefer help and guidance? Some people trust their doctor to make all the decisions, and some want to share in the decision-making process. When you talk to your doctor or someone close to you about this issue, you'll create a clear path to your decision-making process.

Have you been in a strong position in your past where deciding seemed impossible? Try to make a comparison and find out what factors you have considered that helped you in determining the solution for the best outcomes.

What are your expectations from treatment? Sometimes, your options are minimal, and sometimes, you have none. But sometimes, your situation enjoys various valuable options. Understand those options, along with their side effects. One major decision to make if surgery is necessary is to compare the new you to your lifestyle. Will you be content with your new look?

Despite what your doctor or anyone else tells you, focus on your desires and what's best for you. There are many things you know that no one else knows, and the treatment you are receiving may affect those things. You know the potentials that serve as the basis for what happens next.

Do you remember the ton of questions you had in your mind about your treatment? Write them down and prepare yourself to ask your doctor. You need to inquire about various aspects of your disease, including the possibility of your cancer coming back (recurrence) or the likelihood of developing second cancers resulting from the specific treatment you are about to have. The information is overwhelming, so give yourself time to organize your life for your benefit.

Deciding on goals: Now that you have set the ground rules concerning your expectations to help you make the most suitable treatment decision, you must decide on a target. Choosing what you are pursuing regarding treatment can help you constrict your treatment options. Do you wish for a cure, stabilization, or only symptom relief?

Depending on your cancer type and stage, your treatment goals are one of the two leading general purposes, either curative or palliative (chapter 5). To be more specific, goals can be to produce a cure, control cancer, or only to provide you with comfort. Knowing whether your treatment is curative or palliative is crucial and will play a significant role in the decision-making process.

Every cancer patient dreams of a curative treatment. If there is a slight possibility of a cure, take this route. Since this is your wish, you may endure more adverse short-term side effects in return for a chance at a possible recovery.

If your cancer is at a later, advanced stage, or if previous treatments were unsuccessful, you may not have an option of a cure. Here, you may want your doctor to control cancer instead of aiming for a cure. Different treatments may attempt to shrink or stop your cancer from growing temporarily, but again, you may not be ready to endure the side effects of harsher treatments if this is your intention.

Choosing the comfort route is appropriate if your cancer is at an advanced stage where treatment was unsuccessful or if the doctor informs you that there is no hope for improvement. You and your doctor will work together to ensure you are free of pain and other harsh symptoms. In the general sense, curative treatments should eliminate cancer; they will slow, stop, or remove it. Palliative treatments cannot cure cancer, but they can manage symptoms and side effects and focus on the quality for the rest of your life. These goals are often unclear.

In each of the goals, doctors will have considerations. Since in curative treatments the goal is to return you into healthy living, the doctor recommends more aggressive therapies. And although they can have significant side effects, they optimize the likelihood of a cure. Most times, those side effects would be short-term. Effective curative treatment could enable you to return to a healthy life and give you the peace of mind to work hard at improving the outcomes.

Your values and goals will help determine what treatments are best for you. You don't have to make a choice and stick with it. You may change your mind during, in the middle, or even before you start treatment. But you must learn the consequences of such action before you proceed with it. Sometimes, stopping treatment can have a substantial risk to your future health. [R32]

Establishing communication channels: Clear and effective communication with your doctor and the health-care team is a top priority at every phase of your cancer journey, especially when trying to decide on the best treatment option. Let the doctor know everything about you. Don't keep secrets related to your health. The more he or she knows about you, the more they can help. If you don't understand something, ask again and again until you are comfortable with the answer. If you feel you cannot communicate with your doctor, try to bring someone else who can help with communications. You can always record your conversations with your doctor to review, and it's still helpful to take notes.

Getting a second opinion: Doctors are error-prone and don't know everything. Mistakes, although rare, can happen in any medical setting. They may be specialists in their perspective fields, but their experiences may differ. It's always helpful to go back to your first doctor and discuss the new findings of the second, even the third opinion, in order to compare the results. Similar findings by all doctors is a sign that you should follow their advice and recommendations.

What if all the views conflict with each other? What if the doctors' recommendations about many aspects of your cancer differ? This dilemma can increase your confusion and even add to your list of worries. Here, study the individual results and seek help from your primary doctor and ask him or her to aid you in understanding the contrast between the reports and to guide you in the right direction.

Your doctor may provide you with statistical figures about your chances of survival, chances to become disease-free, and progression-free survival rates. These figures are only numbers; they help the doctor predict what *may* happen in your cancer situation as compared to the already researched statistical data.

Statistical numbers may or may not apply to your specific case, but it gives you an idea to help you decide on what treatment is the best for you. Statistics can also help with knowing the side effects resulting from each treatment and their impact on the general population—but can never be case-specific. They're only tools to help you with general findings.

KEEP IN MIND

While you are trying to decide on the best treatment options, always keep in mind to take your time. Although cancer is a time-sensitive matter, taking a little time to figure out the best treatment options with fewer side effects won't disrupt the process of decision making and won't affect the outcomes of treatment. It may reset your thoughts toward making the best decision with the best results.

This period is a milestone in your cancer journey. You may feel isolated from your surroundings since you are preparing yourself to decide on a complex subject. Never imagine that you are alone in the decision-making process. Your primary doctor, oncologist, members of your health-care team, friends, family members, and other cancer survivors are around you and eager to offer their professional and friendly help. All the eagerness to provide support and compassion is at your disposal. It's there to pave the path for you to make the best decisions possible for your situation.

Although the next chapter, "Discovering Resources," is read after you complete your initial treatment, I recommend that you also read it before you start treatment, when you are exploring your options. Besides providing you with literature about the avenues you could undertake after you complete your treatment, it also presents you with information about exploring the best health-care resources to find the best fit for your treatment choices.

CHAPTER EIGHT

DISCOVER RESOURCES

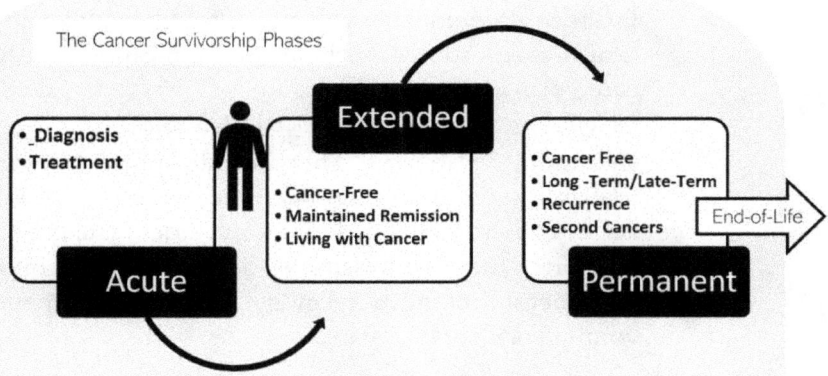

You are preparing to transition into the extended phase

You are in the acute phase and have just completed your initial treatment. Your future health and the specific outcomes are not clear to you or to your oncologist. You may suffer from side effects of the treatment you just had, and that impacted your life. To continue with your journey, you must minimize these effects by finding the appropriate resources to guide you through the adjustment and adaptation processes.

You are exhausted and uncertain about the future, but congratulations on completing the most challenging period of your journey. This time after treatment requires adjustments to the new environment. Many cancer literatures to teach you how to adjust are available in abundance. Select your resources according to your health situation needs. Finding the right resources to help you manage your cancer will make your cancer journey more pleasant and less painful. The main resources are:

- Health-care resources. They include family members, close friends, health-care providers, and health-care facilities. Required tasks and skills related to activating health-care resources include communicating with health-care providers, coordination of services, identifying psychological and psychosocial resources.
- Community resources. They include spiritual, social, and transportation services. Required tasks and skills to activate community resources include managing social support and addressing social or environmental challenges. Joining a religious community depends on your beliefs.

Exploring the new case-specific information is supervised by your oncologist and the health-care team members and depends on your health needs after the treatment.

Your participation in discovering resources depends on your desire and the need to activate part or all those resources. You have had your diagnosis and treatment in a health-care facility that might have or have not been your best choice. You are at liberty to continue with your existing oncologist and health-care facility if you are satisfied with their services. If you are not satisfied, you should start searching for a new oncologist and health-care facility to help you to self-manage the rest of your journey.

The specific information that you choose to enhance your self-management skills is a personal matter that can vary over time as you create a solid structure, optimize your self-management skills, and as your illness and subsequent needs change. You may have to eliminate some of them and gain others, should you need to steer away from obstacles and to fill in the gaps that may arise.

Although self-management is an interactive process, individuals differ in their ability and willingness to take a role or to let others take part in managing their illness. For example, older adults with a chronic disease rarely want their children to assume the burden and the responsibilities of caring for them. This chapter will cover some of the crucial resources that must be researched to assist with executing your future wellness plan while living with cancer.

HEALTH-CARE RESOURCES

These are your health maintenance assets, including the medical professionals who performed your diagnosis and delivered the bad news to you at the medical facility. Health-care resources can also include nonmedical personnel such as caseworkers, volunteers, various assistance advisors, and even the hospital's administrative personnel, where all these people will assist you in every step of your journey. Creating and maintaining a positive relationship with your health-care providers is crucial, and ignoring relationship-building can produce disastrous results.

Before you maintain an adept and productive relationship with health-care personnel, you must search for a suitable doctor willing to accompany you throughout your cancer journey. Excellent past professional experience, place of employment, and recent successes in similar cases to yours might be signs that your choice is appropriate. It is always beneficial to investigate the doctor through multiple channels. So how do you find the most suitable provider, including the health-care facility, to lead the efforts regarding your cancer situation?

The rest of this section may seem similar to previous passages, but, on the contrary, it resembles a new start of your self-management process. You must ask yourself the following questions to determine whether you should proceed with reading this section;

- o Are you pleased with your oncologist and health-care facility where you underwent your treatment, including communication, convenience, and availability?
- o Do the results of your treatment agree with the pre-treatment period expectations dictated by your oncologist?

Remember, complete results of the effect of treatment may not be possible immediately after completing therapy. And, sometimes, the outcomes of treatment don't agree with prior expectations. But the substantial variance in expected results may dictate that you seek another oncologist to explain such a difference. If you answered yes to the questions above, then skip the rest of this section. If you answered no to either question, then continue reading.

Choosing the oncologist: You are not comfortable with your present physician. Doctors are not alike, and sometimes, finding the *right* doctor could mean the difference between life and death. Also, locating your chief oncologist is the first crucial step to managing your disease. You'll be required to perform a complete professional and even personal background assessment on the one you choose.

The general practitioner you saw before your diagnosis might have referred you to an oncologist, a specialized cancer doctor. It's the specialist who will influence every aspect of your cancer care, so you must do your research when choosing the right one for your cancer.

There are dozens of resources to help you find oncologists, including the American Board of Medical Specialties, the American Medical Association, and the American College of Surgeons. Choose a few names of a list of specialized physicians from the places listed above and call for further advice to strengthen your efforts. Your type of cancer may require work with more than one kind of oncologist (medical, surgical, or radiation). The choice of an oncologist depends on your cancer and the plan you have for the immediate future.

Upon choosing the right oncologist who possesses experience with treating your type of cancer, proceed to the next step to inquire about their participation in your health insurance plan, and adjust your search. Your insurance company will be a vital source of information concerning your specific cancer if they cover the cost of treatment and maybe other aspects of the disease, such as clinical trials or complementary therapies.

Now, examine the doctor's credentials by researching their past advanced training and experience with cases like yours, and confirm that he or she is board certified. Always inquire about the length of practice and the successes they had in treating your type of cancer. Get references on their past patients so you can contact them, if possible. Ask questions about the office staff and their experience. Find out little details, such as office hours and availability after hours, and how they would be involved with your care. It's even beneficial if you can get the information you are seeking through references by asking family, friends, and those who received treatment for the same cancer. The next step is choosing the *right* health-care facility.

Choosing a health-care facility: An excellent place to begin your search for the health-care facility is through accredited cancer treatment centers. The National Cancer Institute's (NCI) Cancer Center Program has over sixty centers. Also, contact the American Cancer Society to inquire about cancer centers in your area and whether they offer any types of recommendations. While searching, pay attention to the services provided by cancer centers and learn about the distinction between them.

All cancer centers meet specific standards and fall into two categories, cancer centers and comprehensive cancer centers. Most cancer centers deliver care for people with cancer. Some only perform laboratory research. Comprehensive cancer centers perform the same primary functions as cancer centers, but they also have specialists from different medical disciplines to plan, evaluate, and take care of you.

The National Cancer Institute, NCI, also offers information about the National Clinical Trials Network, once recognized as cooperative groups. These vast networks of researchers, doctors, and other health-care professionals carry out clinical trials throughout the country. There are national organizations that also offer accreditations for treatment.

The American College of Surgeons (ACS), through its Commission on Cancer (CoC), has accredited over 1,500 cancer programs. CoC treatment centers offer many services, including diagnostic, treatment, rehabilitation, and support services. The Joint Commission evaluates general health-care programs. It provides performance reports for thousands of its accredited programs and organizations. Locating the most suitable treatment facility equates in its importance to finding the most suitable oncologist for your cancer.

The methods of priority search between an oncologist and a treatment facility differ from one patient to another. Some individuals find the oncologist and then the health-care facility, most likely the one where the doctor works. Others locate the facility and then search for a doctor. The search depends on many factors, such as the patient's financial status, insurance coverages, the patient's place of residence, and ease of transportation between the facility and the patient's location. If you choose a doctor first, he or she can help you find the most suitable facility. Regardless of the search's starting point, always try to discover the most appropriate entity, while still taking into consideration all the factors involved in the search process.

Similar to choosing a doctor, your choice of a health-care facility for your type of cancer should focus on how much experience the center has in treating your type of cancer and their successes and failures. How valuable is their support system for you and your family members? Will your care team be available for you during holidays and weekends? How close is it to your home or office? Do they offer clinical trials you wish to be involved in? Inquire about transportation help, in case you need it.

The next step is to discover whether you'll receive your medical care in an outpatient or inpatient setting once you choose a treatment center. Although your treatment setting is often determined by the severity of your cancer situation, other times, you may select your treatment's location. The choice of treatment setting depends on personal factors like your financial situation and whether you can afford hospital stays or whether your insurance covers it.

Other elements that can be factors in determining your choice are your family (children, school) and your job situation. For inpatient care, you remain in the hospital, where they will monitor you during treatment and recovery. Outpatient treatment does not cause a hospital stay.

PSYCHOLOGICAL RESOURCES

Although psychological trauma varies in its intensity as you progress through your survivorship phases, you must try hard to contain it due to its negative influences on your progress through the continuum. Emotional changes could increase or decrease after finishing treatment compared to the emotional trauma you may have experienced at diagnosis. Receiving professional care to treat anxiety, depression, and distress after completing your initial treatment is vital for your future well-being.

Discovering psychological resources depends on the urgency of your emotional and mental needs. For changes in your psychological status as you travel through the cancer-care continuum, a new collaboration between you and your medical care team may be necessary to stabilize you. The intensity also varies for different individuals, who demand and new methods of interventions.

As you learned earlier, when patients move beyond the diagnosis phase into intensive treatment, they experience more intense psychological distress and anxiety. Suffering is at its highest levels during the diagnosis phase. Pre-existing levels of distress can be present even before diagnosis. If those patients don't seek therapy, their level of distress remains high, whereas patients who arrive at their diagnosis with lower levels of stress acclimate to the diagnosis and treatment. It's essential to understand the relationship between a cancer diagnosis and the level of psychological distress at any point in time. According to studies, the prevalence of psychological distress does not vary considerably across the survivorship phases, except for the terminal phase.

Neglecting to manage or control changes caused by cancer or sustain normal life activities leads to distress that can reduce the quality of life and may produce poor clinical outcomes. Doctors recommend early screening for distress, done by a specialized counselor, before treatment starts. Rescreening may have been essential at some critical points of the treatment and may continue after completing it. Patients who show moderate-to-severe signs must pursue related resources, such as a clinical health psychologist, social worker, chaplain, or psychiatrist.

The National Health Institute, the National Cancer Institute, the American Cancer Society, and the American Psychological Association are always available to assist you and answer your questions and refer you to the proper channels.[R35]

SPIRITUAL RESOURCES

For some patients, spirituality and religion can be a significant factor in their well-being. They may help patients find a more profound meaning to life and enable them to cope with the disease. It's a hidden strength that some patients resort to during these difficult times.

Spirituality and religion may have different meanings, but sometimes they're used interchangeably. Some define religion as a set of organized beliefs and practices connected to established groups such as Christianity, Islam, and Judaism. Spirituality is a set of behaviors characteristic of the individual, and a sense of inner peace, purpose, and the meaning of life. It's the relationship people have with a force or power beyond themselves that helps them feel connected and enriches their lives. Patients may think of themselves as religious or spiritual or both.

Many cancer patients would identify themselves as spiritual, but not necessarily religious, experts say. Cancer may enhance spirituality in some people. People who are not religious may pursue spirituality and a relationship to a power outside themselves following the diagnosis. Often, people come back to the religious traditions of their childhood. Others may find comfort in a new approach, such as meditation.

The contrast between spirituality and religion diminishes when people face a challenging situation such as cancer—unifying hopes and goals in the sense of gaining strength to stand up to such a dread disease.

"Spirituality is a chance to be reconnected to God, a religious tradition, and a community that provides hope and strength for the cancer patient," says Rev. Deborah K. Davis, director of field education at Princeton Theological Seminary, who was a chaplain at Princeton Medical Center in New Jersey for many years.

Often, cancer patients report that they feel alone because they believe that no one can know their pain.

"Chaplains practice what is called *compassionate presence*, where they make themselves available to help people with cancer feel more connected to another human being, and perhaps to God, during this part of life's journey," explains Barbara Klimowicz, assistant director of pastoral care and chaplain at Fox Chase Cancer Center in Philadelphia. "When I talk to a patient, we talk about being alone in a crowd. They may have a lot of support from family, friends, and community, but they still can feel alone, in the middle of the night, when everyone goes home, you are alone with your thoughts, and you lean on God," she says.

Specialists say that religious or spiritual practices can assist you in adjusting to the consequences of cancer and its treatment. Patients who depend on their faith or spirituality encounter enhanced hope and optimism, liberty from regret, higher fulfillment with life, and emotions of inner peace. Patients who engage in a religious tradition or are in touch with their spirituality are more compliant with treatment and live a much healthier lifestyle. Studies show that spirituality can have a substantial effect on the quality of life by contributing to your physical health through decreased anxiety, depression, anger, and feelings of loneliness. It's shown to influence reduced drug abuse and alcohol consumption. It also contributes to lowering your blood pressure and controls pain and discomfort.

All cancer patients want a cure. If it isn't in sight, they may search for emotional recovery and often wish this healing could come from their spiritual relationship. They desire to find meaning in their lives and their existence, and they search for a sense of support. Decisions about the end of life have a sizeable spiritual component.

"Deciding what you'll do or not going to do has a lot to do with deciding what comes next, if you believe something comes next and you are hopeful, then it may be easier for you to let go of futile treatments," says Davis.

Anger comes with cancer. It's at its heightened level when starting the cancer journey. It dissipates as you travel through the cancer survivorship phases, but it doesn't completely disappear. Spirituality is rarely comforting at the beginning, at the time the patients hear of the diagnosis. For some people, a cancer diagnosis has the opposite effect on their sense of spirituality, where anger can become a factor for detachment from faith and religion. You get angry with God for giving you cancer and think God is punishing you.

This reasoning will make it harder to cope and can lead to apparent spiritual distress. It may hurt the outcomes of cancer treatment. If the situation reaches the point of doubting God, if you are a religious person, then it's recommended to seek spiritual counseling. Experts know that your feelings at those moments are expected, and they can be recognized and managed. Expressing emotions of shaken ideology to someone who may be capable of helping rejuvenate faith, or even comprehend your anger and doubts, can be therapeutic.

Your doctor and the rest of the health-care team know of religion and spirituality issues. They have expertise in discussing this topic and listening to you and can refer you to the most appropriate counselors for help. They understand that each patient has unique spiritual needs based on cultural and religious traditions and upbringings, and they know that these beliefs have a substantial impact on patients' attitudes toward cancer and the challenges ahead.

Pastoral services in hospitals are there for a reason. Ask for a chaplain if you need to and if you think you'll gain comfort from such an event. The chaplain is an educated individual who cares. He will make you feel better through praying and being around you.

Spiritual practices that may help you cope with your cancer and its treatments include praying with someone else who is close to the patient's heart, meditation, and being with someone who shares similar religious and spiritual values. Reading about religion and faith, reading from holy books, admiring God's creations and nature, and, sometimes, joining religious groups or groups comprising individuals who share similar trauma in their lives can produce pleasing outcomes. Research shows that, although religion and spirituality may not affect the result of the disease, they provide the patient with a better quality of life through self-satisfaction and hope.

Faith is a universal word that can mean complete trust in a higher power. Different people may have different views about this subject, but for the sake of this book, I will define faith as the ultimate belief in God. A cancer patient's trust in a higher power gets stronger as they travel on their path through the continuum.[R36]

SOCIAL RESOURCES AND SUPPORT

The National Cancer Institute defines social support for cancer patients as a network of family, friends, neighbors, and community members available in times of need to give psychological, physical, and financial help.

Isolating yourself from your surroundings can trigger a chain of adverse psychological effects like stress, anxiety, and depression. The answer to this issue is to initiate social interactions with your surroundings. At these critical times in your life, you need to interact with people daily to share values and experiences and enjoy each other. Positive interactions are crucial for social development. These social interactions mean that you are not lonely, sad, or depressed. People around you can take away most of your worries through creating and improving social programming. There are many organizations for special needs that give advice, but none of which provide the hands-on help that facilitates real socialization.

Through proper social resources, cancer patients can develop confidence, develop various skills to help manage the disease, make more friends (hence more support), promote physical activities, help ease negative emotions, and reduce the risk of depression. The unification and the association between perceived social support and psychological change show a definite connection following cancer treatment.

A reliable social support system can help you manage your cancer treatment and day-to-day life. By seeking the support of family and friends, you can limit isolation. Find people who have shared similar experiences in the past—patients, caregivers, even friends of someone who had the same cancer experience. Invite people of all walks of life to share in managing your disease. Sometimes, just talking to people about issues not even related to your disease help your situation by making you feel cherished and miles away from isolation.[R37]

You are ready to put your research to the test. Your health has changed, and you have discovered the abundance of resources to help observe your new health needs. This time is when you must try to implement strategies and adapt to what you have learned through discovering your case-specific resources. The next chapter, "Observe Your Health Needs," will help you adjust to the new environment after treatment.

CHAPTER NINE

OBSERVE YOUR HEALTH NEEDS

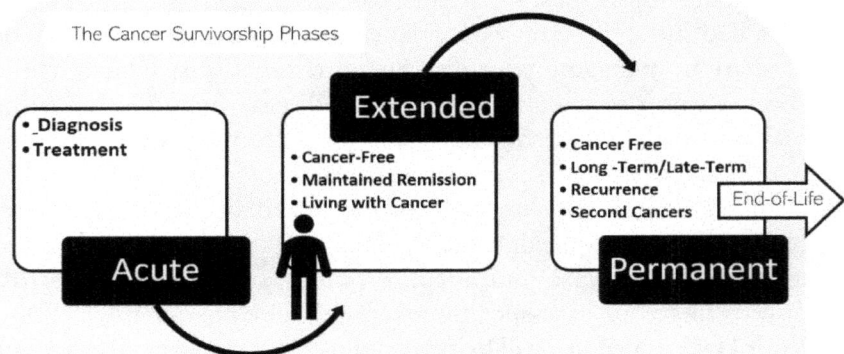

Observe and adapt to the new environment after treatment

You are in the acute phase. Your health requirements have changed after treatment, and you are dealing with side effects, some severe. You have learned about your specific cancer and how to deal with the various consequences by gaining case-specific resources. Before you can transition into the extended phase, you must observe and adapt to the new environment of your health needs by changing your lifestyle.

This period of your journey is essential in the sense that there is a new you. You may have had surgery, chemotherapy, radiation therapy, or some combination of treatments. If you had surgery where parts of your body were altered in a visible area, then your psychological status may be at its heightened state, and professional intervention by a specialist may be necessary. You'll experience a multitude of side effects after receiving treatment, ranging from mild to severe. Now, you must observe your new health needs and adjust accordingly. New health requirements depend on your current cancer situation and the results of the treatment.

Andrew H. Miller, MD, Director of Psychiatric Oncology at the Winship Cancer Institute at the Emory University School of Medicine in Georgia, says, "Most cancer treatments, and cancer itself, can activate the immune system to release inflammatory cytokines. Inflammatory cytokines are chemical messengers released from immune cells that signal to increase or decrease inflammation. Research has shown that inflammatory cytokines can enter the brain and affect many of the brain circuits and chemicals involved in depression, anxiety, fatigue, and impairment in memory and concentration."

You have encountered the words *stress, anxiety, depression, nausea,* and many other similar words in all chapters of this book. It's the ugly reality of cancer that these symptoms can always be your companion at each phase of your cancer journey. On the bright side, most of these psychological and physical symptoms are treatable through counseling and medications.

You can't separate cancer from these devastating words. All the side effects will be enhanced while you are undergoing treatment, and they decrease in intensity as your progress on the continuum. In this chapter, I will cover the side effects of the regimen and what you can do to ease them, how to observe and adapt to your new health needs, changes you may have to undertake to transition to the extended phase successfully, and how to sustain those changes.

YOUR CURRENT PSYCHOLOGICAL STATE

Completing treatment feels like a graduation. You have been in a hard place and endured the anguish that accompanied you during the past few days. Your emotions could be enhanced, depending on your personality and on the results of the treatment. Despite the outcomes, there is a new environment, and you must adjust to it by changing your daily routines. Health adjustments require knowing your present state after treatment.

Now, you must meet with your health-care team, including your oncologist, to discuss the results. Some of those results may be obvious to you since there are characteristics of your emotional and physical feelings, but some others may not be so obvious because of the complexity of your medical situation. Your doctor will clear the path for you to make you understand the complete results, so you can proceed with the adjustments to sustain your progress.

You might be a prisoner of your fears because of negative thoughts. You'll wonder whether cancer has vanished, or if some cells are still in your body. You'll want to know if it's coming back, how soon, and whether your past treatment would have been a reason to cause another cancer that will make you experience the agony again. Remember that no two individuals are identical, so you may encounter emotional changes that are unique only to you and may differ from someone else's, even if they had similar cancer and had the same treatment. This fear may produce anxiety, depression, and distress, where professional counseling is of utmost importance.

General emotions of worry may also include fear, anxiety, and concerns about physical appearance. Feelings of sorrow include sadness, depression, grief, denial, and guilt. They stem from blaming yourself for having cancer and the confusion about future uncertainties, anger about how the disease affects your life, and emotional numbness because of shutting your feelings down for a while. Spiritual distress occurs when you search for a new meaning for life and what it offers you.

You must discover and observe the source of your emotions to manage them. Adjusting to feelings takes time; some survivors need help to change to strong emotions after they finish cancer treatment. Often, your cancer experience will need less of your attention as time progresses. If you are experiencing positive emotions, it could be because of the discovery of new personal strengths and deepened relationships with loved ones, and you are excited about the future.

Some survivors proclaim a sense of gratitude and revived wonder about the positive things they experience. You are ecstatic to be back home, and your loved ones are happy to have you again. You are thinking about now, leaving the future for later, and have developed a sense of self-satisfaction and pride.

PHYSICAL STATE

Noticing a pimple on your face in the morning may turn a life upside down for a teenager. Now imagine that you wake up from surgery only to find you are missing a breast (mastectomy), or that you cannot be intimate with your partner anymore because of prostatectomy (prostate removal).

Physical disfigurement of any sort will influence your outlook on life. Physical disfigurement is made up of two parts. One is disfigurement visible to others, such as a big scar on your neck. The second is disfigurement that is not visible to others—for example, losing a breast.

Sometimes, losing part of your body to surgery can also affect other bodily functions. For example, losing your foot may oblige you to walk with crutches for the rest of your life. Others may affect how other organs in the body function, such as causing heart or lung problems.

Physical changes can lead to intense psychological distress that may need professional counseling. These changes affect you in a way that depends on many other factors, including your whole personality, spouse and family, coworkers, and the public.

Remember that some physical changes may be temporary, such as losing your hair. Sometimes, hair loss could be permanent, such as in areas that are directly affected by radiation. Cancer treatment does not always cause hair loss. The intensity of changes may also depend on your age, gender, and cultural background.

In more details, some potential changes may be scars from surgery, surgical modification of body parts, weight gain/loss, skin changes such as redness of some areas of the skin—itching, more sensitivity, or pain in the treated area, enlargement of the breast, lymphedema (swelling of the arms and legs), and changes in sexual functions.

Body-image concerns are legitimate worries for cancer patients when they affect self-esteem and psychological health. If this is a severe issue for you, if it affects your feelings about returning to work and going back to your usual daily routines, then it is helpful to refer to counseling and support groups at your local cancer center. In certain instances, reconstructive surgery can take care of certain physical deformities. Diet and physical exercise may help resolve concerns. Control of lymphedema can decrease the swelling associated with this health condition. Counseling may be necessary for some cases of bodily changes, if your superiors at work implement some modification that may concern you, such as reducing your pay rate, hours of work, or perhaps changing your physical location at the office for any reason he or she might have.

MAKING THE ADJUSTMENTS

Your next step during this challenge of adapting to your new health needs is to implement effective methods to familiarize yourself with your unique health demands. Your focus will be on recovery, but do not expect too much right away, the road to a new comfortable life may be filled with obstacles, some substantial. Although this process may take time, it is possible to attain hopeful results if you are confident and determined. It is natural to experience significant mood fluctuations, such as depression and optimism.

Ultimately, your inner strength and resilience allow you to endure this experience, sort through options, and determine the pathway of your journey via the difficulties that lie ahead. Reliable coping techniques cause the ability to recognize the circumstance, think through alternatives, consult with those with expertise, and gain the support of others. Ignore no types of changes that might occur despite how minor you may think they are. You will have follow-up appointments with your doctor or members of your health-care team to check on developments or progress and to discuss issues or changes you may experience. Sometimes, going back to normal like you were before the treatment may happen fast, but some people may experience ongoing side effects and may have to adjust to a new routine. If it is necessary to make a few adjustments, then start with changing a few of your lifestyle habits.

Perform research on available complementary and alternative therapies to help you reduce your stress (chapter 4). They can help to lower the side effects of chemotherapy for some people. Many people discover that complementary therapeutic approaches can help them experience a stronger mental capacity to deal with chemotherapy and its side effects. Doctors can use many of these therapies "risk-free" next to the conventional techniques and medicines. You may also wish to try complementary approaches, such as meditation or visualization, or gentle massage, to help you feel less anxious. Many hospitals provide complementary therapies together with standard care. Despite what your choices are, always allow yourself time to readjust.

By now, you are eager to return to a regular daily routine, and good health is at the top of your agenda. You start thinking about your long-term health to enjoy many years of quality. The recommendations offered in this chapter are like those given to anyone else who does not have cancer but wishes to maintain good health. Some of them are exercising, eating a well-balanced diet, sleeping well, enjoying yourself, and reducing stress. Stop smoking and reduce alcohol consumption. Change your present lifestyle to a better one. Following the steps below can have added benefits to improve the quality of life and smooth the transition into the permanent survivorship phase.

Exercise

No one underestimates the power of physical activity for cancer patients who need the added strength. Performing guided physical exercise can speed up your recovery. The benefits include increased strength and endurance, less depression and anxiety, reduced fatigue, improved mood, boosted self-esteem, less pain, improved sleeping habits, and lowered risk of cancer recurrence.

Start a short exercise routine and work your way up to spending more time performing an activity; walk instead of running, take the stairs instead of the elevator, and even perform light exercises while you are sitting down. The American Cancer Society recommends that cancer survivors perform physical activities for at least 150 minutes a week, including strength training at least two days a week. Gradually, you will find out that more exercise makes you feel even better. Do not get discouraged if your fatigue is keeping you from exercising—do what you can, and take small steps until you reach what you desire. If you feel you cannot maintain physical activities, it is okay. Give yourself more time. Do not exceed your abilities; do what you can and remember that rest is also vital to your recovery.

Some studies suggest that exercise may contribute to reducing cancer recurrence and the risk of dying, although the evidence that physical activity can decrease the chance of dying of cancer is preliminary. The proof of its rewards to your heart, lungs, and other body systems is considerable. Implement your guided physical activities as prescribed by your doctor or therapist and report any changes to your health-care team.

Balance Your Diet

Consuming fruit products and veggies and whole grains is always an excellent choice for healthy individuals, and it is necessary for cancer patients. When selecting your meals, the American Cancer Society recommends that cancer survivors:

- Choose healthy fats, including omega-3 fatty acids, such as those found in fish and walnuts.
- Eat at least 2.5 cups of fruits and vegetables every day.
- Select proteins low in saturated fat, such as fish, lean meats, eggs, nuts, and seeds.
- Opt for healthy sources of carbohydrates, such as whole grains, beans, fruits, and vegetables.

By combining all the recommended foods above, you ensure that your body is getting enough vitamins and nutrients to continue having a healthy lifestyle. Research had not proven that specific diets prohibit cancer from coming back, but it is always a good idea to eat fruits and vegetables. Avoid taking supplements unless your doctor or your certified oncology nutritionist approves of such a measure. Your doctor will assign a multivitamin plan that won't harm you or enhance the adverse side effects of treatment.

Control Your Weight

Being overweight can be harmful and can lead to many medical complications, even in nonpatients. You may have weight fluctuations during treatment; some patients may lose weight, where some others may gain a little. You might need help from your oncologist or nutritionist for ways to control it. You may be referred to a certified cancer nutritionist specializing in cases like yours to come up with a plan to take care of your weight issues to achieve the goals needed to sustain good health. If you need to gain weight, your nutritionist will come up with specific ways to make food more appealing to you. Weight loss could result from nausea, vomiting, and pain. Your nutritionist, who will develop a nutritional plan to balance the loss in weight, can control all those side effects.

Cancer patients who need to lose weight must take a precautionary measure and perform the process gradually, only two pounds (about one kilogram) a week. Regulate the number of calories you eat and harmonize it with exercise. It can be a challenge, should the need arise for losing a substantial amount of weight. In this case, do it in small steps and stick with the plan.

Rest Well

Resting most likely involves sleeping. Cancer patients, after treatment, may have problems sleeping. A multitude of factors affects your sleeping habits like stress because of certain medications you are taking.

Sleeping well gives you a break from your surroundings that may produce negative thinking and induce stress. Physical rest gives your body the change to rejuvenate and become refreshed to make you function at your best when you are awake. Sleeping also can boost cognitive skills, improve hormone function, and lower blood pressure.

Avoid the many factors that prohibit you from sleeping like consuming caffeine before bedtime. Regulate your sleeping habits, and do not stay up late at night watching television for too long or socializing with your family members or friends for a lengthy period. You can also make it a habit of exercising two to three hours before bedtime. Do what you must do to produce a specific environment to help you sleep, but don't sleep excessively, as this may make you more tired.

Stop Smoking

According to the Mayo Clinic, smoking causes cancer by damaging the cells that line the lungs. When you inhale cigarette smoke, which is full of cancer-causing substances (carcinogens), changes in the lung tissue begin almost immediately. At first, your body may repair this damage. But with each repeated exposure, healthy cells that line your lungs are increasingly damaged. Over time, the harm causes cells to act abnormally, and cancer develops.

Quitting smoking reduces the risk of cancer and other smoking-related illnesses such as heart disease, stroke, cataracts, diabetes, tuberculosis, and many others. Find out a fascinating timeline of what happens to your body starting at the first minute and for a duration of the first fifteen years of quitting smoking through the American Cancer Society website (cancer.org).

Quit smoking if you are a smoker. Abandon the habit once and for all. The most notable and immediate effect on your body *when you quit* smoking is that your carbon monoxide (found in cigarettes) levels will return to a more reasonable level. When you smoke, this chemical lowers the amount of oxygen in your blood by replacing oxygen particles with carbon monoxide particles. When you quit smoking, your oxygen level in the blood is elevated to its usual level, giving nourishments to tissues and blood vessels. Quitting now could also decrease your possibility of cancer recurrence and lower your risk of developing a second primary cancer.

Stop or Reduce Drinking Alcohol

Drink alcohol in small amounts or quit altogether. For healthy and balanced adults, this means one drink a day for women of all ages and men older than age sixty-five, and up to two a day for men age sixty-five and younger.

Alcohol possesses health advantages in some people; for instance, consuming a drink a day can minimize your risk of heart disease. It also enhances the likelihood of certain cancers, including those of the mouth and throat. Even though it isn't clear whether drinking alcohol can trigger cancer recurrence, it can raise your risk of a second primary cancer. Weigh the risks and advantages of drinking alcohol.

Reduce Stress

It is difficult to reduce your stress if you have a complicated cancer case, but it is possible with professional counseling. Although the concept that managing stress improves chances of cancer survival lacks scientific proof, using adequate coping strategies to deal with stress can improve your quality of life by helping relieve depression, anxiety, and symptoms related to cancer and its treatment. Learn relaxation and meditation techniques, join support groups, exercise, and keep positive interactions with people you love.

Keep a balance in your life and maintain well-being. Some people elect to exercise; others choose to relax. You are the only person who recognizes your body's needs. Meditate, rest, sleep, swim, cook, walk, eat right, watch your favorite shows on television, and go to the theater. Do what you feel will take your mind away from your illness. Reboot, edit, and re-edit yourself. [R38]

TRANSITIONING INTO THE EXTENDED SURVIVORSHIP PHASE

You are about to depart this difficult period of your acute survivorship phase and enter the real long-term self-management phase of your journey. It's time to transition into the extended survivorship phase, where your cancer prognosis can be less ambiguous. Now you know the extent of your cancer and the many challenges you must prepare yourself to tackle. It's appropriate and recommended that you consider a few things while you're transitioning into the extended survivorship phase to ensure a smooth transition. Your future well-being depends on the way you handle your cancer from this instant forward. You realize at this point that transitioning after cancer treatment comes with its own set of physical and emotional challenges. Your doctor, members of your health-care team, your family members, and friends are still around you. You'll manage your situation on your own since you'll have decreased supervision from your health-care team. You must learn how to take those steps almost alone, but remember that help is always available. Here are a few things you could achieve while transitioning out of treatment and into self-management of your cancer as a chronic condition:

- o Organize yourself and write any new changes or developments so you can discuss them with your doctor at your follow-up appointments. Never ignore the more significant changes; they may show more severe problems. The sooner your doctor investigates the issue, the faster he will repair it.
- o Your doctor and the health-care team will not be beside you in the same way that they were when you were undergoing treatment. You've developed a bond with them, and you may think you're alone upon leaving the hospital. Have a positive

attitude and know they're busy helping others, but that doesn't mean that they aren't there for you should you need them.
- Be prepared to experience unexpected side effects that can occur for various reasons. Your new lifestyle habits and the intensity of the treatment may have influenced these changes. You must learn how to manage these new side effects so they won't become obstacles between you and your new life.
- Find the most suitable support groups and specialized support centers. Joining support groups is vital at every phase of your survivorship. But it's essential at this current position (while transitioning into the extended phase) because of its inherent nature; although you have had lots of input when deciding on treatment options, your doctor and the health-care team have done most of the work. Now you have significant decisions to undertake concerning your future and finding your new normal; hence, it helps to join groups of patients who've already walked your path. They can improve your situation by offering advice strengthened with knowledge and compassion. Don't underestimate the power of specific-case support.
- Always hold on to your loved ones and caregivers and friends; they are the people that stayed beside you; they are your central coping and support systems.
- Perform activities that will make you forget about your illness, even for a short while, and have a positive attitude. It always helps to be optimistic about future events.
- Investigate and study the details of your follow-up care plan by discussing it with your doctor and remember: each patient requires an exclusive wellness plan unique to his or her situation.

You're doing great. Welcome to the extended phase of your survivorship journey.

THE EXTENDED PHASE
LIVING THROUGH CANCER

CHAPTER TEN

CATEGORIZE YOUR CURRENT HEALTH IN THE EXTENDED PHASE

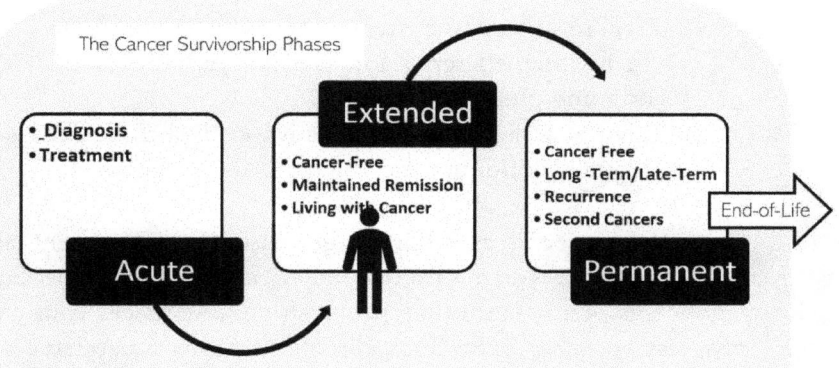

Transitioning into the extended phase of your journey

You're in the extended phase. Upon entering this phase, you and your doctor know your current health situation and the extent of your cancer. For example, the category of your current health is cancer-free, in maintained remission (either full or partial), or living with the disease as a chronic (ongoing) illness. Knowing your category allows you to proceed with the most proper wellness plan specific to your health status.

The extended phase of the survivorship can also be called "living through cancer." A few days or weeks after you complete active treatment, your oncologist will schedule you for an appointment to layout your care plan. This period starts your extended survivorship phase. Your current position on the continuum is a measure of your progress so far and will be explained to you by your health-care team. It is also a period of watchful waiting. The effects of the treatment you just completed are the focus. Recovery begins, and it focuses on the physical, emotional, and psychological effects of the treatment. Most likely, you'll be sent home to continue the journey while help is always available should you need it.

Now you must know your current health status by finding what category you fall under in the extended survivorship phase of your cancer journey. The extended period is comprised of three classes:

- You're cancer-free (treatment-free remission), or
- In maintained remission (staying cancer-free because of ongoing therapy), or
- Living with cancer as an advanced chronic illness that requires continued treatment.

This chapter serves as a knowledge base of your current health situation. It enables you to predict the *near* future of your cancer. Remember this period is the watchful waiting time where your cancer can progress, or not, in various directions. You must have some patience and allow the situation to settle for a few more weeks to pinpoint your precise position within your journey.

CANCER-FREE: TREATMENT-FREE REMISSION

Ignore how doctors define the term *cancer-free* for a moment and enjoy hearing the word *free*, celebrate and hope for the best. Cancer-free doesn't mean that your cancer is gone; it indicates that there are no signs of the disease in your body. The only way to know if you're cancer-free is when a few years have passed after treatment with no warnings or symptoms. However, this situation can't be adequately categorized as "cancer-free" because we can't be sure that there are no cancer cells still lingering until you've passed the test of time.

According to the National Institute of Health (NIH), if someone remains in complete remission—meaning all signs and symptoms of cancer disappeared—for five or more years, some doctors may say a person has been "cured." Having had cancer puts you at a higher risk of recurrence compared to healthy individuals who never had cancer because of your exposure to chemotherapy drugs or harmful radiation.

The American Cancer Society notes, therefore, doctors will rarely say a person is "cured." Instead, they may say things like, "Cancer doesn't show on the scan" or "I see no evidence of any cancer." Usually, by two or three months of treatment, a doctor can tell how a person's cancer is responding.

You're cancer-free or in remission. Remission differs from a cure; it means that you're showing little or no signs of cancer in your body—their disappearance is evident through examinations such as MRI scans or blood tests. Remission isn't a cure, so you still must see your doctor. You may have to take certain medications for weeks, months, or even years to maintain remission.

There are two types of remissions: partial and complete—neither of the two means that you are cancer-free. Complete remission implies that all signs and its symptoms disappeared, and medical tests show no proof of cancer existence in your body. Partial remission means that treatment has killed off most of your cancer cells, but analysis shows that you still have some cancer cells in your body. Your tumor has decreased at least to half of its original size or stayed the same. To categorize cancer as being in remission, it either doesn't grow back or remains the same size for a month after you complete treatments.

Getting into remission depends on your cancer, stage, side effects or risks of each treatment, age, cultural background, or other health problems. When cancer comes back if it comes back, it's called a recurrence. No one knows when it may occur, it typically returns within five years.

Being in remission is a good thing since you start showing a decrease in or even total disappearance of signs and symptoms of cancer. Besides taking lower doses of cancer drugs or hormones to keep the disease from coming back, there are things you must do to stay where you are at or even improve to full recovery. Your wellness plan prepared by your oncologist will have plenty of advice to help you maintain good health. Proper execution of the plan is important in order to sustain progress.[R40]

MAINTAINED REMISSION

Maintenance remission is staying cancer-free because of ongoing therapy, treating cancer with medications, following an initial round of treatment. Maintenance therapy may include chemotherapy, hormone therapy, or targeted therapy. Its primary purpose is to prolong the patient's life and not to cure the disease. The goal of treatment during maintained remission stops current cancer from getting worse through stopping or slowing down its growth. Both types of remissions, full and partial, require maintenance therapy during the extended phase with the possibility of administering it to the patient for a long duration. It isn't a new concept in cancer treatment, but it is more common nowadays compared to the past for a variety of reasons, including introducing new cancer drugs and the constant improvement of therapeutic technology.

Nowadays, cancer drugs are abundant compared to the past. Many of these drugs aren't being used for initial treatment but are suitable for maintenance therapy. Advances in the pharmaceutical field made it possible to create cancer drugs with less harmful effects than old medicines. Also, the use of these drugs makes it longer for cancer to come back if it recurs. It's an established medical fact that maintenance therapy can help extend the lives of people with certain types of cancer but doesn't work for all kinds of cancers. It might include drugs from the first treatment plan and may involve the use of another drug or a combination. Maintenance therapy makes use of traditional chemotherapy drugs where some drugs are more effective than others. This therapy is useful after treating some types of leukemia and early-stage breast cancer.

Maintenance therapy is also used after initial treatment for several other cancers, such as advanced lung and colorectal cancers and some kinds of lymphoma. The therapy can take weeks, months, or years depending on the situation, drugs used, how well it works, and how long you can endure side effects of such treatment.

Some people feel safer when receiving maintenance therapy; however, others think they aren't cancer survivors if they're still getting treatment. Either way, maintenance therapy is an integral part of many people's treatment and recovery plans.

Maintenance therapy doesn't come without baggage. Although it can keep cancer from coming back and may help slow its growth, it also comes with various risks and burdens, including experiencing more side effects. It can even get expensive since you must see your doctor more often to receive the treatment. This inconvenience is an added cost that some patients can't afford. Investigating this issue before attempting this treatment is always beneficial. Resources to perform such a study are available in abundance through your caseworker, your insurance company, your oncologist, and the rest of the health-care team members. [R40]

CANCER AS A CHRONIC ILLNESS

In third place in the extended phase is the chronic category. Doctors call it "a chronic disease" (an ongoing, advanced disease where continued treatment is required). Here, the tumor is considered an incurable illness like diabetes and heart disease; it lasts more than three months. Some cancers, such as ovarian cancer, leukemia, and some lymphomas, are considered chronic. Many others that have metastasized are also regarded as incurable, including breast or prostate cancer.

Chronic cancer, like other incurable illnesses, can be controlled and treated; it may not grow or metastasize while receiving treatment. The treatment may shrink it where, in this case, you can stop the process until it comes back again, even though it will always be there. Cancer during the chronic phase may be stable when scans or tests show that it is not changing. Anything can happen to cancer during this phase; it can go into complete or partial remission. However, doctors can't speculate how long it stays in remission. Some types of cancer have the tendency of recurrence and remission such as ovarian cancer. Often, this repeating cycle of expanding, shrinking, and stabilizing can mean survival for several years were managing it as a chronic disease is workable. If cancer comes out of remission, it is said to have progressed, like recurrence, but with variance in intensity. If it develops during or soon after treatment, it may mean that a different therapy may be needed.

If cancer comes back, then you will have to start all over again (chapter 6, "Understand Your Diagnosis"). During the new diagnosis, the hope is that your emotional and psychological status is less severe than when you learned that you have cancer the first time. You might have to go through the same treatment as when you first started or through different ones—it all depends on the type of cancer, stage, and progression. Navigating treatment options (chapter 7) starts all over again for the upcoming round of treatment if there is one for your situation. It isn't recommended to ask to halt treatment even at your current status.

Treatment can be in the form of chemotherapy, and there are two ways to use it: 1) Maintenance therapy, given on scheduled regular basis where chemo may help slow or stop the spread to prolong life, and 2) When cancer is active again or when it changes. However, cancer cells can become resistant to chemo after a while; the tumors that keep returning don't respond to therapy as the first tumor. As an example, if cancer returns within a year or two of getting chemotherapy, it might be immune to this chemo, and another drug may be a better choice. Physicians will state, "You've already had this drug, so we need to try another one." This action can mean that they think you've received all the help you could from a particular drug and an additional one will better kill the cancer cells since it functions differently.

Your doctor won't choose a particular drug because of the risk of an immediate side effect or because you have had that drug before. For example, some chemo drugs may cause heart troubles or nerve damage in your hands and feet. It would not be suitable to continue with giving you the same medication since it would risk making those complications worse or even lead to permanent damage.

Your oncologist can't estimate the length of the treatment at the beginning. It depends on many factors such as the designated treatment plan, duration of time between cancer recurrences, the aggressiveness of your cancer, your overall health and age, your tolerance, how well you respond to treatment, and the treatment used. You can expect your health to deteriorate, and the doctor will give you an idea of what to expect.

You may ask, does the treatment help? For some situations, it helps; for others, it doesn't. You may also start wondering about the usefulness of continuing this therapy. You may think it's painful to continue if it's becoming an obstacle between you and enjoying life, which can lead to you feeling bad all the time. Stopping treatment is your decision, but always inquire about future happenings should you take that route.

You might arrive at your decision to stop treatment when you had several therapies that didn't help halt the cancer; this suggests that your cancer is resisting all treatments. Weigh the limited advantage of a brand-new treatment versus the potential downsides and the stress of getting therapy and the unfavorable side effects that go with it. Talk with your family members and cancer-care group about your intentions and what you can get out of therapy. They can help you make the most effective choice on your own. Depending on your situation, consider supportive care in the form of palliative care (chapter 5), or if your case is degrading fast, find hospice care (chapter 5). Alternative and complementary therapies (chapter 4), clinical trials (chapter 3), and counseling are also choices to consider. [R41]

COPING IN THIS PHASE

The first few months after cancer treatment are a time of change. When you're coping with cancer that doesn't disappear, it may seem like you're stuck in this change. You don't know what to expect or what's most likely to occur next. Coping with cancer isn't about "getting back to normal"; it is about what's normal now. People often claim that life has a new meaning or they look at things in different ways. Everyday tackles a new definition that holds unexpected events.

Your brand-new "normal" may include making adjustments in the way you eat or changes to a new lifestyle, things you do, and your resources of support. It may imply connecting your cancer therapies to your job, family functions, and your daily routine. It will suggest making therapy part of your everyday life—that you will always have for the rest of your life. Cancer will affect everything you do with no exception; it controls your actions and become your permanent companion.

Repeated cancer recurrences, often with shorter periods between remissions, can become discouraging and exhausting. It can be more disappointing if cancer cells never go away. The concern of whether to keep dealing with cancer that doesn't vanish or returns is legitimate. Your choices concerning proceeding and continuing with therapy are personal and depend on your demands, capacities, and dreams. There's no right or wrong decision on how to handle this period of the illness, and there's no universal formula to follow to make the most suitable choices.

Having incurable cancer doesn't put you beyond hope or help; you may live with a disease that can be treated and controlled. The extended phase may have a few side effects that may stay with you depending on your health situation:

Uncertainty: All these changes and challenges that seem impossible give rise to skepticism about what will happen. There's no specific way to deal with uncertainty. Try to control what you can, and ignore what you can't control. Some individuals say that putting their lives in order makes them feel much less afraid. Being associated with your health-care team, searching for your "new normal," and making modifications in your way of living are some of the things you can regulate. Also, establishing a day-to-day timetable can offer you more power. While no one can control every thought, some say they've resolved to not dwell on the fearful ones.

Sadness: It's normal to feel sad when you learn you have incurable cancer. This unhappiness might not disappear, even if you live a very long time with the disease. You may experience grieving the loss of what you thought would be your future. These events are hard for anyone to handle without emotional support.

Pain: Pain can affect a person psychologically and physically. It can interfere with daily tasks. It requires time and power to adapt to these substantial changes in your life. Many people find it helpful to have individuals they can talk to about all these points. If no person comes to mind, you could see a counselor or a support system to assist you with your pain. Doctors can always treat physical pain with medications.

If cancer has already spread, the hope is that it can be stopped or slowed down, but the hope may change if treatment ceases to work. This difficult period is the time to prepare family and loved ones who will be left behind, for telling them what they have meant to you and what you wish for their futures. This kind of link can enable a great closeness to the people you adore.

You may wish to plan the end of your life, where you invest your last days in doing what you want. It can ease the burden of uncertainty your loved ones may have about what to do and what you'd want. Your clear plans can be a considerable gift to them and help them be at peace with the tough selections they might have to make when you can no longer say what you want. Despite what your current health is, you must start an initial-care plan unique to your situation. The purpose of such a scenario is to lessen many emotional and physical side effects of your treatment.

YOUR INITIAL SURVIVORSHIP CARE PLAN

This period is when the survivorship plan begins, and it serves as the first care plan you'll encounter during your journey. It contains advice and recommendations by your health-care team (nutrition, lifestyle changes, and recommendations for follow-up care), aiming at optimal health. Your oncologist and the health-care team prepare your case-specific survivorship plan according to the overall analysis of your current situation. It will set the ground rules to transition you into the permanent survivorship phase.

Having gone through treatment, you wish to return to normal, the way you used to be. It's a fact that you may not go back to your usual routines, and you'll have to search for a new normal that meets present and future needs specific to your health and wellness. To achieve your new status, you need constant monitoring by your health-care team. This care provides you with the knowledge and support to adapt to positive lifestyle changes.

The care or wellness plan prepared by members of your health-care team (nutritionists, oncology nurses, oncology physical therapists, and other members) supervised by your oncologist serves as a professional guide to steer you into healthy living. It also includes recommendations on how to continue to get the care and provides risk identification and reduction through health promotions, prevention, and screening. It provides management and monitoring for side effects of cancer and its treatments, scheduling of screenings for possible recurrence, referrals for any follow-ups necessary, and resources for continued care. A survivorship care plan can also include information to help meet your emotional, social, legal, and financial needs.

A survivorship care plan, also called a follow-up care plan, can't be underestimated as a vital tool to ensure your future well-being, it tracks survivors from a wellness perspective. Advances in cancer research are leading to an increase in cancer survivors, where individual concerns are unique. Of the approximate ten million cancer survivors today in the United States, about seven million have survived for five or more years; and these numbers will continue to grow. Since each cancer situation is different, awareness, education, and guidance are critical. An individualized and personalized care plan focuses on each survivor, taking into consideration family history, geographic location, cultural and spiritual backgrounds, and more essential elements such as the type and stage of cancer, your age, and health issues. A survivorship care plan contains the following features:

Treatment summary: Includes details about the diagnosis such as date, type, stage, location, progression, and histology of your cancer. Names of all your health-care personnel, including your primary care doctor and the treatment facility, are also a part of the care plan. The care plan will detail the treatment you received, such as chemotherapy, including the doses and drug administered, radiation dosage, surgery, or any other form such as immunotherapy or even if you have received any alternative and complementary therapies.

Follow-up plan: This part of the care plan is comprised of recommendations for ongoing care, such as visits with the oncologist, surveillance testing for recurrences, and management of long-term effects. Part of this section of the plan will be reserved for health promotions comprising lifestyle habits or changes. It offers recommendations concerning diet and exercise specific to your case and detailing harmful practices such as smoking or drinking alcohol excessively.

You must collect a substantial amount of data concerning your current and past health situations. Details of resources, surveillance methods, and patient's services must be organized to prepare for the most proper recommendations. The wealth of information you have collected, and the unique experience you are enduring, are preparing you to find and accept your new self. Recognizing yourself as a new person isn't complete without trying to adapt to the new health environment. Adaptation will award you the power to continue into the permanent phase where you manage your cancer as a chronic illness. The next chapter contains an ample amount of information to prepare you for adapting to your new health requirements.

CHAPTER ELEVEN

ADAPT TO YOUR NEW HEALTH NEEDS

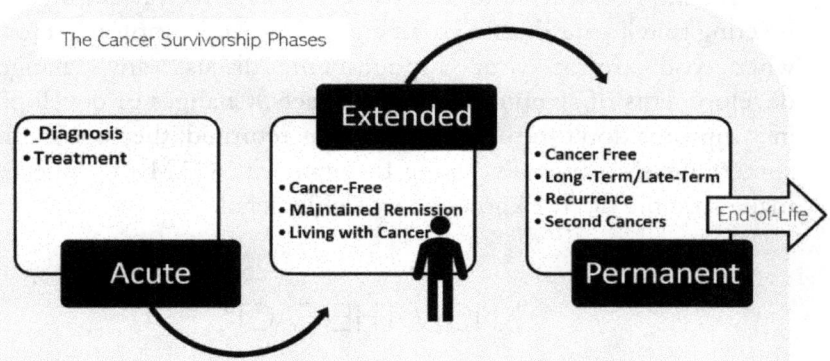

Final preparations to transition into the permanent phase of your journey

You're in the extended phase. Your present health situation and the future of your cancer determine your wellness program according to the oncologist's understanding of your cancer situation. Execution of the plan comes in the form of adjusting to a new health environment, including performing more changes in your lifestyle. The future outcomes of your cancer depend on your willingness to adapt to the changes.

Adapting to the new life after completing treatment depends on where you are on the cancer continuum. Each category in the extended phase, detailed in the previous chapter, requires its own set of psychological and physical adjustments.

This chapter outlines a wellness approach for each health category. Although these strategies of health adjustments may be specific, they may not be the correct strategies for your cancer case.

During this period of health adjustments, you may also face new decisions like what to do when treatment doesn't stop or when it isn't helping anymore. By now, you have a wellness plan specific to your situation. Don't settle for the information in your case plan without understanding all the details; ask many questions to make clear of all aspects and features.

It's important to note that you don't have to wait until your next meeting to tell your doctor about any changes or symptoms. However, when you are at your appointment, discuss any changes or developments of symptoms or side effects. Changes or developments in symptoms don't mean that cancer has returned; they could arise for something else. If you've gone through with CAM or clinical trials, make sure the doctor knows every single detail.

KNOW THE FACTS

This period is an excellent time to have another look at your lifestyle. Even small changes to your environment and surroundings, including your place of residence and the people you associate with, can be beneficial for your future. This change is significant if you think your surroundings may impose even the slightest danger to your health.

Several of the feelings you may experience could be favorable or unfavorable. The positive thoughts and feelings you're experiencing could result from knowing you've completed the treacherous period of the treatment and a little beyond. They could also be attributed to knowing that you're going home to unite with your loved ones and friends or going back to work and have a healthy life again. Negative thoughts and feelings may develop because of the fear of cancer recurrence. Being in maintained remission or living through cancer as a chronic illness as opposed to being in complete remission may trigger and contribute to your negative thinking. The various medication the doctor prescribes to help maintain your health situation may also have side effects that add to your negative outlook.

You may have a short-term or long-term effect in the after-treatment period. Symptoms and side effects unite in the period after completion of the treatment. Most patients will experience physical weakness, such as fatigue, and others will experience a difficult period of anxiety and depression. If you had surgery that affected your physical appearance, you might experience varying degrees of stress at work or in public. Your sex life might have changed or delayed while you were in treatment, or you may even still suffer the consequences for a long time and, sometimes, permanently. You may also deal with complicated financial matters. You may not have your hair. No matter what your thoughts and feelings may be, you must adapt to the new reality to attain the best hopeful outcomes of your situation.

Dr. Larissa Nekhlyudov is a general internist who works with cancer survivors at two Harvard affiliates, Brigham and Women's Hospital, and Dana-Farber Cancer Institute. She acknowledges that cancer survivors have a lot to encounter. "Once you've had your final chemotherapy infusion or swallowed the last pill, you may face a new set of challenges—monitoring yourself for signs of recurrence, getting recommended follow-up care, adjusting to the long-term effects of treatment, adapting to normal life, and working to stay in good health," Dr. Nekhlyudov says.

So, does a general strategy exist to ease all those negative feelings altogether? Although it depends on many factors, including your personality and the harshness of the treatment experience, adjusting to the new environment takes time, and it becomes easier to deal with feelings. Many changes will occur. Some may require more attention and hard work, and some will be irrelevant. Often, you'll need less time to focus on your cancer experience, which will help you adjust.

NEW PSYCHOLOGICAL ADJUSTMENTS

Psychological turmoil impacts patients and their families. The most important effect is depression resulting from the accumulated stress that started at the diagnosis meeting. The ability to cope with stressors comes with varying intensities, predictabilities, or unpredictabilities with varying levels of vulnerability.

Most psychological problems appear insidiously, but specialists can normalize the impact. They are often not acknowledged or dealt with promptly. This negligence occurs regardless of the reality that psychiatric conditions are now recognized to take place in approximately 30 to 60 percent of newly diagnosed patients with various types of cancer. Neglected depression has been shown to have multiple unfavorable outcomes. Besides the psychological suffering because of depression, developing anxiety has significant effects on morbidity (condition of being ill or unhealthy) and perhaps mortality in cancer. Proof suggests that resolving psychosocial, psychological, and physical signs early in the cancer trajectory, through using palliative care or mental interventions, might affect survival outcomes. Comorbid anxiety (more than one disorder in the same person, for example, social depressive disorder, and major depressive disorder coexisting together) results in a decline in quality of life. This situation can serve to increase the level of sensitivity to discomfort, interaction troubles, caregiver burnout, increased risk of suicide, longer duration of hospitalization, and a decreased expectation of survival. The most substantial psychological issues that may accompany cancer patients through this period of the cancer journey are feelings of worry, sorrow, and confusion, and they are addressed below.

Feelings of Worry

Feelings of worry may present in a troubling form, including fear of recurrence, anxiety, and concerns about physical appearance. Every patient fears recurrence with the absence of signs and symptoms. People react to changes with their physical appearance depending on the results of surgery. It depends whether changes are visible, for example, losing hair, a noticeable scar on your body, or physical changes the public doesn't see, such as losing a breast or a certain bodily disfigurement.

Your feelings of worry will fluctuate depending on many factors, most notably, your current environment. Are you in a peaceful place according to your standards? Is it quiet like you want it? Are there any people around you who increase your anxiety? Can you get rid of them and connect with others who give you support and create a comfortable environment for you? Only you can answer these questions. Changing your environment and surroundings to your liking will reduce your feelings of worry.

Do something soothing like learning deep-breathing techniques and try yoga. Find healthy ways to deal with pressure and to calm yourself down. You must think positive and abstain from overthinking. You can control your thinking through imagining a pleasant moment of your life or by occupying your time with activities you love or even being with a dear family member. Abstain from things that can make your worry worse, such as consuming caffeine, and follow a nutritional plan to give you the energy you seek. If your feelings of worry are causing anxiety and impeding your life, you might consider professional counseling.

Feelings of Sorrow

Feelings of sorrow can accompany you at all phases of survivorship, but with varying degrees and intensities. They include sadness, depression, grief, and guilt. Even at this point in the journey, feelings of sorrow present themselves in almost every cancer patient. Depression results from a long-term situation of stress, and it's caused by or becomes worse with chemical changes in the brain. Grief could be a long-term effect after treatment, no matter what your position on the continuum—grieving about a healthy life you once had. Besides deep sadness, the grieving process may also include stages of denial and anger before one can reach full acceptance of the loss. Guilt is blaming yourself for having cancer because of things you've done in the past, and it is conventional and natural among most cancer patients. You might feel guilty that you survived cancer, but others did not, or you might feel guilty because of the burden you may have on someone else because of your illness.

Can you do anything about the feelings of sorrow? You bet; it's possible to rid yourself of these negative feelings. You must try to accept the fact that there's a timetable for healing from sorrow, so give yourself some time to heal. Another helpful way to heal is to be close to someone you love, like your spouse or a loved family member, including children. People close to your heart can bear a significant burden and take away some of your sorrow without you even realizing it. Again, to manage any negative psychological issues such as sorrow, it's always recommended that you perform an activity to keep your mind occupied with something positive such as picking up a new hobby or traveling to a place you love. Eating healthy and exercising are also useful when you deal with negative feelings. Perform meditation and get soft supervised massages to calm your body and mind. You owe it to yourself and your family to try hard to liberate yourself from negative feelings of sorrow.

Feelings of Confusion

Uncertainty, anger, emotional numbness, and spiritual distress may produce confusion in many patients, especially when you're feeling unsure about the future condition of your health; for example, you may be nervous before a medical follow-up appointment. Remembering the day of the diagnosis may also bring out uncertainty. You may have anger because of what cancer has done to you and forced changes to your life. It comes and goes, depending on your cancer situation. Emotional numbness, the experience of no feelings, results from the stress caused after the treatment. You might feel that you can't take it anymore. Emotional numbness causes you to shut down all your feelings for a while. Spiritual distress happens when you search for a new meaning for life, and it's essential to well-being for some patients. Suffering can begin if life becomes very different from your expectations. Some survivors may redefine values and goals during this period of confusion.

These terrible feelings may be new to you in the sense that your life before cancer lacked their existence. Everyone, even nonpatients, experience some of these feelings in their life because of a variety of factors where the intensity of such factors varies in severity, depending on the source causing such feelings. Individuals will experience much confusion because of fear about the future. For example, losing a job that results in financial hardship will inflict confusion about the future mixed with fear, anger, and uncertainty. These feelings will diminish as soon as the individual's problem is solved, such as finding another, perhaps even a better, job. But the situation with each cancer patient is different. They may experience most or all these feelings at the highest intensity, and they might all accompany the patient at the same time.

These feelings are a lot to handle, and adjusting to your new life without some or all these stressors is critical to enabling you to progress in your cancer journey to attain the best outcomes. Although each one of those psychological issues can be considered a standalone mental condition, it's best if you can combine all of them under the same umbrella and repair the problem as one. The process will be complicated, but with the proper professional guidance, the sought-after outcomes are possible.

Although confusion can cause many negative feelings, being confused will also help you grow and change. How would you improve, adapt, and always adjust if everything made sense to you? Start by accepting who you are and who you became after your experience with harsh treatment. Take a deep breath and think about your uncertainty and move out of it; it's a major cause for your sorrows. Focus on what you know and on your feelings to eliminate some obstacles causing your confusion. Any occurrence takes time to resolve; it's a matter of time. It helps to be patient and do your best to combat these feelings. Time will heal.

PHYSICAL ADJUSTMENTS

Physical and psychological elements are analogous to each other after cancer treatment, where physical challenges can give rise to emotional troubles. Cancer rehabilitation specialist Julie Silver, MD, an assistant professor at Harvard Medical School, says the goal for patients should be to find the best physical solutions that go together with emotional healing before accepting the new normal.

Physical and psychological adjustments make up a dual journey as the patient tries to tackle the harsh reality of the disease and search for a "new normal." Several serious challenges face cancer patients after completion of treatment. Some are treatment-related, and others are general because of cancer itself, where some challenges are short-term while others are long-term. The severity of certain physical side effects depends on the treatment and maybe simple tiredness, long-term disabilities related to physical losses, or more tangible issues such as chronic pain. Fatigue, memory loss, nerve damage, heart and lung problems, and a multitude of other physical impairments can add to the problem. Further complications arising from physical challenges could be related to employment and lifestyle changes. While most of the side effects are typical with most patients, fatigue and pain stand out like shining stars. A few treatment therapies for fatigue and pain exist where effectiveness of such therapies rely on various factors including the cancer and the treatment received. The next few paragraphs summarize the most notable side effects.

Fatigue

Extreme tiredness and a constant feeling of being worn out is a significant complaint most cancer patients have during the first year of recovery. Fatigue differs from being tired, and you can't cure fatigue by resting or sleeping. The intensity of fatigue varies for different individuals and depends on the type and stage of cancer and the treatment patients received. Cancer therapy causes fatigue experienced by patients undergoing treatment because of the damaging effects the patient's immune system experiences. According to Macmillan Cancer Support, causes of cancer-related fatigue (CRF) aren't understood. But it's logical to assume that these effects are due to the harshness of certain drugs used and their adverse impact on healthy cells. Other causes of fatigue are related to poor nutrition, anemia, and changes in eating habits. Also, pain can contribute to causing fatigue since it's a source for draining the patient's energy supply. There is no preset pattern for side effects. They can last for a long time or a shorter period, but for some patients, the side effects get better with time. People who had bone marrow transplants may experience fatigue for a long time, which may not improve and becomes a part of life. Fatigue can take over the patient's life where its effects can be noticeable daily, including affecting the ability to perform work at your job and various family functions and daily routines.

Your oncologist understands you might be a prisoner to fatigue. He will provide you with the best wellness plan to lessen your struggle and, for some patients, may eliminate it. Your doctor can recommend various methods to boost your energy, such as drinking more fluids, changing your eating habits to include vitamins and minerals to help you gain extra strength, adopting specific exercise program, taking certain medications, or recommending that you see a specialist like a nutritionist, occupational therapist, or even a mental health counselor. Don't rely on your doctor to solve your fatigue problem; there are many things you can do to gain more energy. Some points I used to mention to my patients when they complained about being extremely tired included the following:

- o **Plan your every daily move:** There are a million things you would like to accomplish either as a part of your daily routine or a part of your life. Write what you need to achieve in

ascending order relative to their importance. Do what you can but lightly.
- **Rest well when your body asks you:** Never sleep for long periods as this may make you feel more tired. Take only short naps whenever your body tells you to do so, and save the long sleeping period for nighttime. Each time you lie down, close your eyes and try to have positive thoughts. If you end up sleeping, then that is what your body wanted. It also helps to listen to relaxing music while resting.
- **Get out for short, light walks:** Short, light walks help your blood circulation without causing exhaustion. Don't run, as this may drain your energy, causing you to feel more tired.
- **Perform light required activities sitting down**: If you must perform specific actions, such as washing dishes, washing clothes, cleaning the counters, do it while sitting down. Standing up while performing certain activities can consume part of your energy.
- **Associate with people dear to your heart**: When you are having fun with friends or family members dear to your heart, you ignore your physical troubles. Being around certain people gives you more motivation and, hence, more energy.
- **Speak with someone who walked your path:** As with many issues you encounter during your cancer journey, speaking to someone who had a similar experience produces tremendous help. What worked for them might not be suitable for your situation, but using some logic always places you in the right spot.
- **Choose how to spend your energy:** Make conserving energy a goal. Plan it and always choose how you spend it. If you think going out to the grocery store exhausts you, then try to ask a family member or a friend to have groceries delivered to you.
- **Join support groups:** Certain groups can be of significant advantage to you. Some group members can advise you on specific issues that you may have missed. You can ask a lot of questions and expect a lot of real answers.

Pain

Cancer pain appears because of tissue damage resulting from chemotherapy or radiation therapy or because of cancer itself. It can also happen when cancer grows and pushes on nearby organs, for example, putting stress on bones and nerves. The tumor can also release chemicals that can cause pain. Cancer pain becomes chronic because of the chronic nature of the disease. All forms of cancer produce pain, with varying intensities among patients. Different patients may experience varying degrees of discomfort, even if they have similar cancers.

Surgery can produce pain because of the removal of cancer in the area of extraction. Sometimes, this could be because of a nerve injury caused by the surgery, or it could be phantom pain because of the removal of a limb or breast. Radiation therapy can cause the pain associated with redness and burning sensation of the skin, along with mouth sores, diarrhea, or fatigue. Chemotherapy causes pain linked to nausea, fatigue, infections, and nerve pain (neuropathy). Strong pain medications themselves can cause further pain issues, such as constipation, nausea, vomiting, and drowsiness. Even weak medicines like aspirin or Tylenol can create an array of physical problems, including damage to your kidney, and cause ulcers and may increase your blood pressure. How one experiences pain depends on cancer type, stage, and the individual's tolerance. There are three main types of pain: acute pain that eases off quickly, chronic pain that stays with you and never disappears, and breakthrough pain when medications are used to treat chronic pain. Other less popular types of pain can be felt in an area away from the actual source of the pain, for example, feeling shoulder pain during a gallbladder attack. Phantom pain is when the patient senses pain in a region of the body that isn't there, for example, feeling pain in your leg after amputation for sarcoma, or experiencing pain in your nipple or your "breast" after a mastectomy.

Not every cancer patient has pain. When the cancer is in its advanced stages or if it comes back (recurrence), chances are pain will increase. The good news is that cancer pains are manageable. Controlling pain is essential to treatment, but how is it treated?

Doctors may treat pain by erasing the source through surgery, chemotherapy, or radiation therapy. If treatment for some pain isn't likely, then the doctor resorts to recommending the various pain medications depending on its severity. Drugs are made up of a few classes; some are 1) weak medications such as those you get from your local pharmacy or grocery store like aspirin, Advil, ibuprofen, and Tylenol; and 2) strong medications, including opioids, for example, codeine, and potent opioids such as morphine, oxycodone, fentanyl, and methadone. Your doctor may prescribe others, such as antidepressants, antiseizure drugs, and steroids if the need arises.

Many people take advantage of alternative and complementary therapy methods to control pain. Acupuncture, massage, hypnosis, and others may help some patients. These unconventional methods, although unproven to help with reducing pain, have helped many patients.

Doctors are reluctant to prescribe strong medication to some patients because of fear of addiction. Sometimes the patients don't mention a pain to their doctors because they fear that cancer is worsening or because of other personal reasons. Some patients avoid taking pain medications for fear that their lives will be taken over by the side effects that strong medicines can cause, such as sleeping a lot, which may lead to missing out on daily routines or not being able to perform well at their jobs.

A specialist manages and controls pain, not your regular doctor. Your pain specialist will study your physical and mental situation before he or she attempts to put you on a pain regimen. Your specialist will give you enough medication to balance your life and perform your routines without interruptions.

FINDING THE OPTIMAL SOLUTION

During my supervision of group coaching and counseling sessions with my cancer patients, I used to combine all their psychological problems as one main issue. At some meetings, patients' groups were comprised of cancer patients of varying ages, sometimes with notable age differences. The outcomes of such designed sessions were expected, especially for the older generation. My analysis showed that older patients were more content with their health situations compared to younger patients. These results were because they believed they'd had long and satisfactory lives and accomplished most of the tasks they'd set for themselves, including raising children, saving money, and so on.

Younger patients, in their twenties and thirties, envisioned cancer as a disease that interrupted their life in every way, where most of them did not even have the chance to get married and raise children or pursue their dreams. It's essential to state that the older generation also enjoys the wisdom and experience that accompany old age.

A general solution to solving all emotional issues that accompany cancer at various phases of a patient's survivorship isn't possible. But it's possible to implement a few strategic factors to at least come as close as possible to a unified solution. Each individual and his or her cancer is different, and the complexity of the disease only adds to the already significant problem of trying to find answers to emotional issues. Hence, a general solution is hypothetical, and it lacks scientific accuracy. Younger patients with an aggressive form of cancer may require a variety of different psychological interventions, such as counseling, as compared to older patients, to aid them in controlling the situation. So, is it possible to at least try to implement a general solution to come close to solving the emotional problems facing patients? It's possible if we apply a few principles of problem-solving, they include the following:

Identify the problem: Before you confront the situation, you must identify its existence. Once that's accomplished, you must determine its exact nature, including all relevant components, such as goals and barriers. Having succeeded so far provides you with a platform for investigating a broad range of interventions and gives you the ability to generate options. This step involves developing a clear problem statement that can be linked to specific goals and objectives. When identifying a problem, consider not only the challenges but also the constraints on opportunities that are preventing the goals and objectives from being achieved. To identify a problem, you must have a substantial amount of data related to the issue you're trying to pinpoint. You already have an abundance of data available to you to pinpoint your exact problem. Should you need any more data, resort to your oncologist or the existing available resources and not-for-profit organizations.

Analyze the problem: Analysis is made up of a set of analytic tasks to enable you to understand a situation. Part of the analysis is to recognize it in a suitable form and to break it into smaller pieces. After examining each element for simplification and getting appropriate solutions, then you can find the common denominator and apply it to the whole situation. Part of the answer to each component is in knowing the goals you must achieve for each element. If you don't see what you're working toward, you will never know when you've arrived there. When applying this knowledge to your cancer situation, you must ask the following questions: How often do you experience all the feelings that contribute to the problem? What are the unique circumstances that caused it and kept adding to it? How long has it been going on? How is it affecting your life? Finding answers to these parts of the whole situation will give you the ability to address each one and combine all the solutions to the entire problem.

Identify decision criteria: They are principles, guidelines, and requirements necessary to help you decide. These are a set of variables to make you identify the critical points to solving your problem. Variables could make up time, quality, experience, efficiency, features, style, convenience, comfort, risk levels, and the best satisfactory results. They help test alternatives and give you a better ability to make choices. You can ignore variables that are common and general to every situation so you can narrow down your options, particular to your specific case. In your cancer situation, it's how you decide when it's time to choose, and the circumstances that may influence your decision are the variables under consideration.

Develop multiple solutions: Sometimes, there is only one solution to your problem, but you may also have various resolutions, so how do you find and choose a suitable solution to the challenge? The method here was like your research when you were navigating for your treatment options; the same applies when trying to find answers to your emotional issues. By now, you recognize that you have a problem and know its extent. You have analyzed it and identified the variables that you may able to ignore, which takes you to the next step to combine all this knowledge into focusing on the most relevant findings. Organize and sort through the results and prepare to find the optimal solution.

Choose and execute the optimal solution: Use the criteria you developed and prepare for contingencies, study the pros and cons of every situation, and consult with others who can help. Never stop at the first solution that makes you feel comfortable, exhaust all the possibilities you have concluded, and perform an accurate comparison before you decide. Execute your optimal solution after you finish your search where the execution of results should be carried out under the careful consultation and supervision of a professional. Consult only with those who possess the knowledge and qualifications to help.

In the next chapter, you will combine all your problem-solving knowledge and expertise and use it to nurture your mind, body, and soul, the last step to prepare you to enter the permanent phase of your survivorship journey.

CHAPTER TWELVE

NURTURE YOUR BODY, MIND, AND SOUL

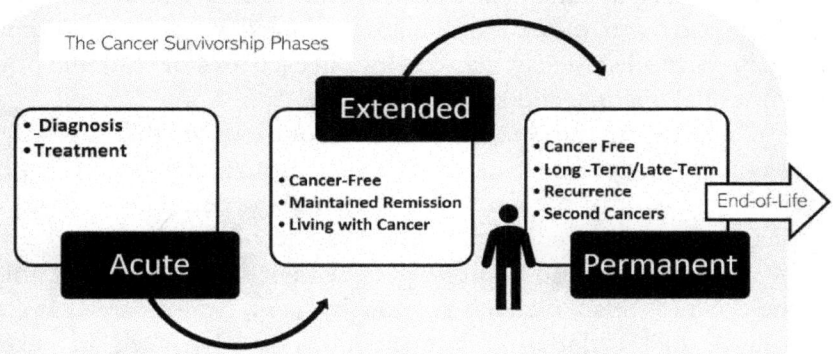

The last step before transitioning into the permanent phase

You're in the extended phase. Now, you will prepare to transition into the permanent phase of your survivorship to implement everything you have learned and combine all the knowledge to nurture your mind, body, and soul as one. This necessary act prepares you to begin an optimal self-management process of your future health according to the category relative to your cancer situation.

Self-nurture is a pre-requisite for self-care that aids in the successful self-management of your cancer. Now is the time to believe that you're worthy of tenderness and able to provide it to yourself through your thoughts and actions. It's the willingness to treat yourself with generosity and protect yourself with boundaries. It's always challenging to change your lifestyle habits to new ones, but the self-nurture process guides you on how you spend your time and relate to yourself and others.

You must know and identify your minimum necessary self-nurture practices, for example, sleeping well, a daily visit to your mother, get rid of your television, letting calls go to voicemail, dedicating time to reading your favorite books, and listening to relaxing music. Nurturing can also arise from more substantial activities such as becoming a patient advocate, volunteering, learning about your illness to teach others, and being involved with your community. Brainstorm a list of activities you love in each area of your life: physical, emotional, mental, and spiritual.

You're about to enter a phase of your journey that may require a massive amount of work where self-nurture can be an important deciding factor of the outcomes. Entering the permanent survivorship phase of your cancer journey is quite an accomplishment.

To maintain and improve your current status, you must abide by the wellness plan dictated to you by your health-care team. Your wellness plan includes recommendations on a balanced diet, exercise, resting and sleeping well, trying out specific complementary therapies, and perhaps a million other things specific to your cancer. All these requirements become a part of your daily life, and you must know how to manage them with precision and dedication. However, would doing so improve your health? Yes, but it also depends on your cancer type and stage, and your present health and attitude.

The next few pages will show you how to go the extra step and become more involved in your cancer to help yourself, and perhaps other cancer patients. You can be an excellent teacher to those newcomers, and they'll trust you even more than their doctors. Knowing they're receiving education and directions from someone who walked their path encourages them to improve their outlook about the future of their cancer. You help yourself progress for better outcomes while assisting others who need you. But before you try to help yourself and others, you must have a positive attitude about the future and unite your body, mind, and spirit as one to work for your advantage.

YOUR BODY, MIND, AND SOUL

Your body's biological complexity is composed of thousands of processes that occur every second—inner intelligence or the spirit coordinates such complex operations. It's a self-regulatory and self-repair mechanism to guide your mind and body. External factors such as carcinogens can harm the body leading to diseases such as cancer. Environmental factors will interfere with the efficiency of these processes, causing a disturbance in the way they perform their jobs, and when the body receives these messages, it will interfere with the self-repair mechanism and predispose us to disease. Techniques such as reflection, pranayama, and yoga exercise (yogic breathing strategies) can bring equilibrium back to mind and body while resolving the great special significance of cancer in your life.

Your body receives the most unpleasant experience of cancer during and after the treatment by experiencing the physical side effects like fatigue, pain, and sleep disturbances, as well as other significant experiences, including chronic pain. Your first line of protection against any illness is your body's immune system. Chronic inflammation in the body can add to the upkeep of abnormal cells; a healthy immune system is necessary to help clear cancer cells. With a durable immune system, the human body can identify and clear itself of recurring abnormal cells after the first therapy. If the body's immune system isn't healthy and balanced, then it can't acknowledge and remove these abnormal cells. By boosting our defense features, mind-body methods can complement whatever therapies you began.

Many mind-body practices have been proven effective in treating the significant side effects of conventional cancer treatment methodologies. Via reflection, we can regulate the discomfort of intense stimulations (a process of pressure, friction, temperature changes, or chemical substances to the skin to lessen or block pain) that the body is sending out, therefore perceiving much less displeasure. Also, meditation has been shown to have beneficial effects on sleep and fatigue in cancer patients, and can also affect pain levels. According to research studies, yoga improves quality of life in breastcancer survivors, including improvement in handling pain. The old technique of pranayama, or breathing methods, has likewise been revealed to have an advantage in cancer patients getting radiation treatment. In a pilot research study, the approach of breathing strategies was shown to reduce sleep disturbance and lifestyle ratings when practiced throughout chemotherapy treatment cycles.

Your mind is the entity that receives and processes emotions. Emotional stress resulting from having cancer or because of the treatment can affect your physical being. It's natural to have a full range of various emotional reactions to the disease, but it's also essential to manage them. Unmanaged stress or suppressed responses can send biochemical signals that put your body in fight-or-flight mode. Because of this interference, your immune system may become suppressed via hormonal and neurological pathways, which can also induce inflammation, resulting in compromised healing ability. Via reflection, we come to be witnesses to the feelings we have, and we access brand-new understandings and analyses of our ability to handle our subjective experiences much better.

Many studies are documenting the benefits of meditation, yoga, and pranayama on anxiety and psychological tension. These mind-body treatments turn around the excitatory and hormone paths that are triggered through stress and anxiety feedback by causing the relaxation response and even shutting off the fight-or-flight paths they've established. They're useful not just to take care of the feelings that turn up with cancer therapy but also to boost lifestyle after treatment.

From a spiritual perspective, cancer can disconnect you from reality and our true nature through disturbances resulting from the many annoying distractions it produces. Spirituality restores your sense of infinite energy, and it's the secret to assessing your most in-depth source of that energy, creativity, and healing. Calmness, resilience, and focus can manipulate challenges. Meditation develops your confidence by tapping into the timeless realm within your awareness. When we nurture our affections through relationships with others, we explore the divine energy that attaches us to all things. The love and help of people around us are causes of strength and healing and can keep us healthier.

Mind-body techniques can be implemented into any course of treatment and throughout your cancer survivorship. It can make your body more responsive to the many changes that occur. You're more receptive to your own self-regulatory and self-repair mechanism. By recognizing cancer from a mind-body-spirit perspective, we can see the value in choosing treatments and methods that deal with both our emotional and physical layers. This recognition accesses our most extensive resource of health and wellness and all-natural equilibrium through daily spiritual techniques.

Depending on your current health situation and the severity of your cancer, you may have reached a point in your journey where you need help to go forward. You're stressed and can't sleep, your appetite is fluctuating, and you're lonely even when you're around people. You resent your life, and a solution must present itself to you before you go into a distressed mode where special professional attention is critical. You have been seeing doctors and specialists from your health-care team for a while now, but nobody can help you. There are several things you can accomplish to get liberated from all the above daily distractions caused by your cancer. I have successfully used the following three tips on many patients. Besides mind-body practices, a few powerful tools to help you detach from cancer are the subject of the next few paragraphs.[R44]

In the introduction to part two, I noted that to succeed in your journey, you must nurture your mind through becoming involved in various activities that serve two primary purposes: 1) to take your mind away from the disease, and 2) to give you the knowledge to ensure the best outcomes for your condition. The main recommended activities are comprised of coaching, volunteering, advocacy, and providing free cancer-resources services.

CANCER COACHING

Part of nurturing your mind is to become involved in the new practices of health-and-wellness coaching. This practice can go in both directions. Either you receive professional coaching to help you with your current situation or you become a cancer coach by taking advantage of a short academic program offered by many well-respected institutions. The field of coaching has been growing as people have become conscious of their health and well-being.

Coaching will help you find the motivation and tools to reach your physical and emotional health goals by allowing you to make better choices that fit your lifestyle. The benefits of becoming a cancer coach include your ability to do the following:

- Establish effective communication channels with your doctor.
- Learn how to pick up the pieces after the damages caused by cancer and treatment.
- Integrate yourself into a healthy level of functioning and well-being. This process is vital in teaching you how to transition from one phase into the other in your survivorship journey.
- Get a higher level of health literacy, including scientific and medical.
- Make you understand health insurance jargon to help you use it for your benefit.
- Gain a thorough knowledge about clinical trials, palliative and hospice care, and alternative and complementary therapies and use them to your advantage.

The benefits of becoming a health coach are unparalleled. You become the absolute pilot of your journey. As a result, your negative emotions will be simpler to repair to focus on recovery with a clear mind.[R46]

VOLUNTEERING

Volunteering has its surprising benefits. The right match can assist you in reducing stress, finding good friends, getting in touch with the neighborhood, learning new abilities, and even advancing your profession. Giving to others can likewise help safeguard your mental and physical health. When you offer essential aid to people in need, worthwhile causes, and the community, the benefits can be even higher for you, the volunteer. Volunteering and assisting others can also combat anxiety, keep you stimulated, and offer a sense of function. While it's true that the more you volunteer, the more advantages you'll experience, volunteering need not involve a long-term commitment or take a considerable amount of time out of your hectic life. Giving in even basic methods can help those in need and enhance your health and happiness.

Volunteering is giving your time and knowledge to others with no expectations in return for your services. Cancer volunteering is an honorable effort, and the benefits are substantial for both you and cancer patients you're trying to help.

Being a cancer volunteer, you're contributing to helping those with cancer. The self-satisfaction resulting from such a gesture is overwhelming. Other benefits of becoming a cancer volunteer may include receiving free training that may help your cancer case. Besides the knowledge you gain from being a volunteer, you'll meet new exciting people and make new friends who can be vital should you ever experience any feelings of isolation because of the effect of the disease. If you volunteer in a hospital or a cancer clinic, you'll encounter many cancer patients who may share similar cancer experiences with yours. Having people who share similar experiences like your own makes both parties share information, and sometimes some of it could be vital and life changing.[R47]

CANCER ADVOCACY

A third example that may have a significant impact on you and other cancer patients is cancer advocacy. It's the act to help improve the lives of people with cancer, including your own. Becoming a cancer advocate is a positive and empowering experience. Advocacy is like volunteering in the sense that many avenues may make up your ambitions. Before you become an advocate, you must choose what branch of advocacy matches your personality and expertise. You may wish to support cancer patients, help raise money for cancer research, make efforts to change public policy, help cancer research through cancer clinical trials, educate people in the community about many advances in cancer and treatment, raise awareness of cancer events, or moderate social media sessions. No matter what you choose, you must develop the skills to do it. There are plenty of resources to give you a jump start with your new endeavor. A simple search will reveal the many resources you can use to become a cancer advocate. An ideal place to begin is the National Coalition of Cancer Survivorship to inquire about joining an advocacy group.

You need not have expertise in a medical branch or cancer patients advocacy to become an advocate. You can act as a liaison between the patient and the research communities and clinicians. Clinicians and researchers grasp the diagnosis of cancer in its medical setting but may lack other talents, such as translating medical terminology into a form comprehended by the layman patient. Patient advocates bring a nonscientific viewpoint to the research process and communicate the patient perspective.

A particular branch of advocacy I see necessary is advocating to improve communication between patients and doctors because of the critical importance of communication. A patient advocate can act as a liaison between the two parties to establish a connection. Advocacy can also come in many other forms, including public speaking, community meetings, writing a blog, and others based on your interest.
R47

PROVIDE A FREE RESOURCES SERVICE

Your experience with cancer made you an excellent teacher. During your journey, you may have spent long hours researching your cancer situation. You have been at many meetings with your doctors and members of your health-care team and a few multidisciplinary professionals. You have endured much physical and mental pain and due for graduation with honors. These events make you a well-experienced and a well-educated individual. Why not use all that knowledge to benefit others who are just starting?

The idea is to establish a free information resource service such as a newsletter, an internet website, a blog, online courses, weekly meetings with patients, speaking events, or any creative idea of your own. By now, you know what works and what's real. Newcomers are thirsty for legitimate, fulfilling, and beneficial information. Cancer patients can't waste time; every minute of every day is precious. Your resources can help cut down on research time performed by other patients and allow them to have more time to execute that information for their benefit. I can't imagine any cancer patient saying no to such a concept. Imagine the self-satisfaction you gain from such an endeavor, and always know that anything you do for other patients might open your eyes to something new that may benefit your situation. Your efforts to allow for genuine interactions with others, some who might have more knowledge than you, can help your situation through collaboration and information sharing.

It's useful to others if you can provide your services while joining community educational sessions. Your involvement in your community is one of the most important projects you can be involved in while sailing through your journey. It can be through holding educational community sessions through a church or school or even giving speeches and offering seminars in various locations. Teach people what you have learned. Nonpatients in the community will be invited to attend such sessions to learn about prevention and early screening. Make them understand that it's a matter of life and death, and prevention is the only legitimate cancer cure so far. [R47]

Having cancer need not paralyze your daily routines or activities. You can still be an active citizen and play a significant role in helping others while helping yourself. This part of the strategy has been placed at the end of the extended survivorship phase while preparing to enter the permanent phase since you're entering the long and lasting self-management period. What this means is that you have already gone through the emotional diagnosis shock, treatment, follow-ups, cancer research, and probable physical side effects of treatment. And now you must use your experience to help you manage your cancer, perhaps, for a long time. The experience makes you a great caring teacher.

The road ahead remains long and scary and demands the same attention from you as every past step. You're about to enter the last phase of your survivorship, where a lot can happen. The main issue you may face is a constant worry about the return of cancer. Recurrence will occur if it's destined to happen, and cancer can strike anyone at any moment. You're ready to transition into the permanent phase of your journey.

THE PERMANENT PHASE
LIVING BEYOND CANCER

CHAPTER THIRTEEN

CATEGORIZE YOUR CURRENT HEALTH IN THE PERMANENT PHASE

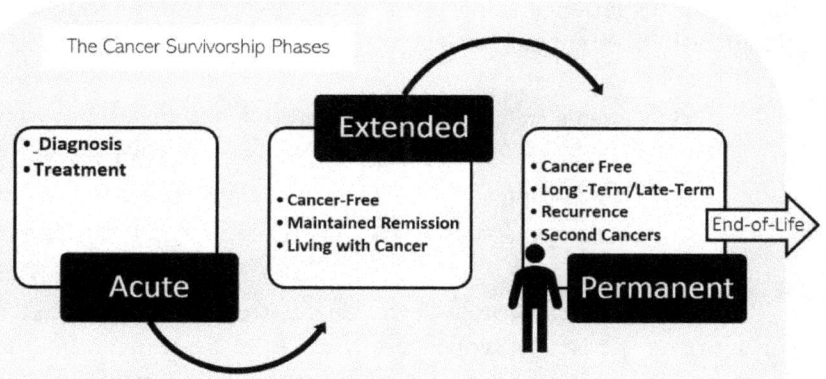

Entering the permanent survivorship phase

You're in the permanent phase. Despite your current health situation, you still have come a long way. In this phase, you're cancer-free, you suffer from long-term/late-term side effects, your cancer came back (recurrence), or you have developed second cancer. This phase requires a new set of health promotion that depends on your *exact* health status. A new case-specific wellness plan prepared by your oncologist may be necessary to help you continue your journey in the best way possible.

You have just entered your permanent survivorship phase. As in the case with all the previous phases, future progress to maintaining a good quality of life demands an ample amount of work and proper execution of your wellness plan.

This phase is when your confidence comes back, your life becomes normal again, and recurrence is less likely to materialize. Long-term effects are the focus, including any challenges that may arise in the form of psychological problems and secondary effects of the treatment.

You may still suffer from psychological, psychosocial, and physical side effects of the treatment, and you may need continued care by a specialist who knows about long-term effects. Two-thirds of survivors may say that their lives went back to normal, but around one-third will experience long-term issues. This phase contains four classifications or subcategories:

- Cancer-free and asymptomatic
- Cancer-free with long-term/late-term problems
- Developing second cancer (unrelated to earlier treatment)
- Developing second cancer (related to earlier treatment)

These are subcategories of the cancer-free status of the extended-survivorship phase. If you were found to be cancer-free in the extended period for the months or even years after finishing treatment, then there will be four subcategories, mentioned above, that serve as possibilities for your future with cancer. Once your oncologist determines your position, you must customize a new wellness plan specific to your current status. Even if you have maintained a cancer-free status up to this point doesn't mean that you're safe from recurrence. The reason behind needing a *new* wellness plan upon entering the permanent phase of survivorship is because of changes in your health requirements and needs, for example, worsening of certain late effects, having second cancer, or introducing new guidelines to continue improving your health while you're still cancer-free or in maintained remission. Your doctor may also refer you to specialists from other medical disciplines to take care of all variables listed in your care plan, for example, a cancer nutritionist, physical therapist, even a spiritual counselor if needed. In the following few pages, you will discover what the four subcategories mean.

CANCER-FREE AND ASYMPTOMATIC

The disease is asymptomatic if you're a carrier for an illness or infection but have no noticeable signs or symptoms. Being cancer-free, without comparison, is the best position in the survivorship stage. A few months or even years have passed by with no signs or symptoms. Routine medical tests can't detect cancer anywhere in your body.

A cancer survivor, despite health condition during the whole survivorship duration, is at a higher risk of recurrence or developing second cancer than nonpatients who never had cancer. It can also mean that the malignancy will never come back where it resolves itself and become benign. During this period, you're still obligated to visit your doctor and go through some tests and scans to ensure that you need no more treatment to maintain your position as being asymptomatic.

Many patients are relieved, but they may feel lost and confused. They'll have many unanswered questions. They're confronting their feelings and wondering about the future while not being able to forget the past. Their recent experience has taught them how to view the future from different angles and the changes they must carry out in their lifestyle to maintain wellness.

Being cancer-free and asymptomatic requires some hard work, like going the extra step to stay sound. Each significant event—like the diagnosis meeting with your oncologist, the start of treatment, completing treatment, or surgery during your cancer journey—is a milestone, and being cancer-free is the best and most memorable one. While each occasion has its own set of mixed emotional, psychological, and physical happenings, for some individuals, it could be celebrating a great accomplishment, and for others, it could be a trigger for a range of emotions, ranging from gratitude and relief to sadness and fear. Accept those milestones as progress forward and know how to use them to the best of your knowledge. Make them the signs to reflect and learn and above all, celebrate. You may need to make more adjustments in your life at this point to keep the progress going, such as creating more friends or changing more lifestyle habits. Try to recognize those milestones where recognition comes in many forms:

Take some private time to reflect. Think about what just happened to you and about the harsh experience you endured and how it affected and changed your life. Share your thoughts with others close to you and come to peace with yourself.

Do something special for yourself. Plan on taking a trip somewhere either alone or with a loved one. Enjoy it and try not to think about your disease.

Help others. Lend a hand to others who share a similar cancer experience with you or volunteer to help them through using the knowledge you have gained. You can help cancer patients who are newly diagnosed, and offer them the expertise you've learned from your cancer experience.

Celebrate. Share your joy with those who are celebrating their milestones. Some organizations host events that may already recognize these types of special occasions, such as annual walks or races hosted by client advocacy groups and not-for-profit organizations. Some hospitals and support centers hold reunions and other events for cancer survivors. Celebrating turning points don't have to include pricey or sophisticated activities. Any activity—such as a walk in the woods, seeing a movie, or getting a massage—can be a unique event if it's something you like to do. Run a marathon and motivate patients and nonpatients. Keep in mind that everyone experiences cancer and its turning points differently. How you pick your unique moment makes your experience special and essential.

CANCER-FREE WITH LATE/LONG-TERM EFFECTS

Cancer problems appearing months or years after treatment are called late-term effects, and patients who underwent chemotherapy are at risk of developing such issues. Testing and treating late effects is an integral part of your survivorship wellness plan.

The late-term effects depend on the cancer and the treatment you've received. No two people are alike, even if both had the same cancer or treatment. Some of these side effects can be controlled with medications. As always, when you take care of the problem in its initial stages, treatment is possible, or it can even vanish it. There are a multitude of late effects affecting cancer patients in the long run, and it isn't possible to cover all of them in this book. Hence, I will pick the most common late effects that many patients may suffer. For patients who experience late effects not listed in this chapter, your doctor knows of the problem, and he or she will treat it. It helps to research your late-term effects specific to your situation as soon as you know what they are.[R48]

Late effects could be mild or severe, where some may improve or go away with time, such as anemia, and some are permanent, including certain types of nerve damage. Various effects occur because of the treatment you received, and they can't be avoided. Medical attention to any new symptoms or enhanced current symptoms is required. Below, you will find specific late effects of the main three types of cancer treatment, including surgery, chemotherapy, and radiation therapy. Your age could be a factor in determining the severity of those long-term effects.

LATE-TERM EFFECTS OF SURGERY

Surgery is one of the leading three cancer therapies along with chemotherapy and radiation therapy, and it's essential in treating many cancers. Not every cancer surgery produces long-term effects. The effects of some types of surgery are minor and may leave nothing more than a little scar, and, in other situations, they could be substantial, for example, when the surgeon removes a breast or limb or even a whole organ. In severe cases such as eliminating a body part or organ, the surgeon does the most excellent job to limit the effects of surgical treatment by balancing and removing all cancer out while removing as little healthy body tissue as possible.

Removing some healthy tissue around the tumor leads to more damage. But it might be necessary to ensure that all (or most) of the cancer cells disappear. Removing healthy tissue causes more severe health effects compared to regular surgeries not related to cancer. Improved surgical methods have helped to lessen the risks, but late effects may still occur. The good news is that not all cancer patients will experience late-term effects from having incisions. Below is a list of some of a few of the most common late-term effects of cancer surgery.

Scarring: Many factors impact the extent of scarring after surgery, for example, the age of the patient, genetics, and the site of the incision. Scarring in older patients is less prominent (the scar doesn't look as bad compared to scars in younger adults), although it takes longer to heal than in younger patients. Genetics is the primary factor impacting healing time for a scar. People with a dissatisfactory family history of scar formation may be at increased risk and decreased healing time. The location also affects healing time and whether the patient should consider reconstructive surgery. Although disfigurements can be invisible to others, sometimes the incision can be in a prominent location, such as the breastbone, or over significant joints. These types of scars can be prone to thick, expanded scar formation in anyone. Surgeons have many methods for treatment, including scar placement, lasers, steroids, and revision, which involves cutting out the whole area and then restoring it.

Lymphedema: It's the swelling of the arms, legs, face, or neck from the buildup of lymph fluid. Surgery can produce lymphedema in cancer patients; it's common because of the removal of damaged lymph nodes caused by surgery. Here, the surgeon may remove lymph nodes near the growth to see if cancer has spread. When lymph nodes are taken out, lymph vessels that carry the liquid from that area to the rest of the body are secured, also, because they're wrapped around the nodes. Taking out these lymph nodes and vessels makes it harder for the lymph fluid in specific parts of the body, such as arms, legs, and neck, to flow to the chest where it can return into the bloodstream. If the remaining lymph nodes and vessels cannot eliminate enough of the fluid, then it builds up and triggers swelling or lymphedema. People with cancers that spread to the lower abdominal area are at a higher risk of lymphedema. Doctors recommend that patients perform light exercise concentrated around the affected limb. This action may encourage lymph fluid drainage and help prepare the patient for everyday routines, such as doing light housework. Other techniques to help with lymphedema is bandaging your entire limb; it encourages lymph fluid to flow back toward the trunk of the body. Massage is also beneficial for treating lymphedema; this technique called manual lymph drainage, which promotes the flow of lymph fluid out of the arm and leg. You must consult with a certified lymphedema therapist before you perform any of these techniques. The therapist can introduce you to other possible case-specific methods to lessen the swelling.

Nutritional problems: Cancer surgery can lead to appetite changes, which sometimes causes weight loss. Changes in appetite can lead to weakness and fatigue, which causes you to eat less and, hence, have less energy. Treatment of nutritional side effects could leave the patient with nausea, pain, and constipation, which are the common causes of appetite changes. Eat small meals or only snacks and try to drink a lot of fluids. Try eating with people close to you to get the encouragement you need to maintain a healthy diet since these people may have a positive influence on you. Create an atmosphere where you're most relaxed while eating, for example, listening to music, or watching your favorite TV show. Eat food high in calories and high in protein like peanut butter, eggs, cheese, nuts, chicken, and an array of other beneficial foods detailed by your nutritionist.

Memory loss: Weakness in concentration and experiencing temporary short-term or even long-term memory loss is another effect of surgery depending on the incision performed. Stress and anxiety, fatigue, anemia, infections, and hormone problems can cause memory and concentration problems or make them worse. Doctors treat memory problems with medications and cognitive rehabilitation. Many complementary therapies, including meditation, breathing techniques, relaxation, and visualization, can also help with memory loss. Performing various brain activities such as reading, word puzzles, and brain teaser games may also help.

Cancer surgery can cause other physical problems, including deficiencies in fighting infection, changes in sexual functions, and fertility issues that can sometimes lead to intimacy issues, chronic pain, and difficulty with speech. These physical issues can open the door to emotional changes, where professional counseling is necessary.

LATE EFFECTS OF CHEMOTHERAPY

Chemotherapy medications disrupt cells of the body that are rapidly growing, for example, those that are related to hair, skin, fingernails, or the stomach lining producing short-lived adverse effects. These include mouth sores, upset stomach, hair loss, or skin rashes. Adverse effects improve as the healthy tissues repair themselves.

Not all chemotherapy drugs have the same late impacts. A lot depends on the type of drug used and, on the dose, and whether its use took place with another kind of treatment. If an organ is damaged, it depends on whether it can repair itself. Some late effects of chemotherapy include fatigue, difficulty with focus and concentration, heart and lung problems, muscle weakness, kidney problems, and hair loss that could be temporary. In the next view paragraphs, I will outline a brief description of the most common late effects of chemotherapy.

Brain Changes: As in the case of some cancer surgeries, memory loss is also possible after chemotherapy. Other problems are weaknesses in concentration and processing information, personality issues, and movement problems. You may have to see a physical, occupational, or speech therapist who can help with these issues. Your doctor may provide you with some drugs to improve your situation, or you may be referred to surgery to reduce or eliminate the problem.

Hearing Loss: Using certain chemotherapy drugs (in specific, cisplatin, and high dosages of carboplatin) can trigger hearing loss, and you must see an audiologist afterword to prohibit a long-lasting hearing loss. You need to have at least one visit with an audiologist after you have finished treatment if you had a cancer therapy that can trigger hearing loss. Depending on the type and dosage of cancer treatment you received, you might be required to see an audiologist regularly.

Heart problems: Cancer treatment can also trigger heart problems, including congestive heart failure, or when the heart muscle is weakened. Because of these heart troubles, you may experience shortness of breath, dizziness, and swollen hands or feet. Other problems such as coronary artery disease can occur when the blood vessels that supply blood and oxygen to the heart become narrow. Chemotherapy drugs can damage the heart or peripheral blood vessels, or cause issues with clotting or blood lipids. It can also cause chest pain or shortness of breath, which is even more notable in patients who had high and direct doses of radiation therapy to the chest that accompanied chemotherapy. This problem needs professional medical attention. Your doctor may suggest a plan to take care of your heart, such as following a balanced diet rich in fruits and vegetables and whole grains, weight control, and exercise.

Bone and joint problems, osteoporosis: Bone problems are a common issue because of chemotherapy. It weakens the bones and causes them to become fragile and fracture easily (thinning of the bones). The good news is that there many lifestyle strategies and physical activities that can improve bone mineral density. An exercise that focuses on postural stability and resistance strength training is effective. Strength training helps prevent falls and improves balance, hence reducing your risk of hip fracture. Joint pain, like arthritis, occurs in the hands, knees, hips, spine, shoulders, and feet and is most apparent after several hours of inactivity. Treatment-related joint pain can be distinguished from the pain that accompanies a recurrence or metastasis because it's a generalized pain felt in multiple places, whereas cancer pain is site-specific. The cause of treatment-related joint pain isn't known. It's essential for cancer patients suffering from bone and joint problems to start a physical therapy program supervised by a certified oncology physical therapist with your oncologist's supervision. Different people with these types of issues need various exercise programs because of factors like age.

Eye problems: Treatment can increase the risk of cataracts, causing eye problems; it's a condition in which the lens of the eye becomes cloudy. Cataracts trigger multiple issues where it affects the whole eye, from blurred or double vision to sensitivity to light and trouble seeing at night. Some chemotherapy drugs can trigger dry eye syndrome, a problem in which eyes don't produce enough tears. Signs resemble feelings as if your eyes are dehydrated or have something in them. Your doctor will refer you to an ophthalmologist to treat your cataract where he or she may have to perform surgery sometimes. In this surgical treatment, an eye surgeon will get rid of the clouded lens and replace it with a plastic lens. You will have local anesthesia and go home the same day. If you get a dry eye syndrome, your surgeon might recommend routine treatment with eye drops or ointments.

Other late-term effects of chemotherapy include lymphedema, urinary problems, early menopause, and developing secondary cancers. The severity of such effects may worsen if chemotherapy and radiation are combined and used for a single treatment or a round of treatments. Unfortunately, in certain cancer situations, the patient may have to receive a mix of treatments to ensure better results where late-effects are enhanced.

LATE EFFECTS OF RADIATION THERAPY

Radiation therapy targets the areas of the body affected by cancer. The effects of radiation only appear in the treated area. Sometimes, treatment may also target healthy tissues to ensure the best results.

Newer methods of radiation treatment help reduce damage to healthy tissues. Treatment is directed to the same area each time.

Radiation rays often scatter, leading to tissues and organs near the cancer site to receive little doses of radiation if this occurs. Effects of radiation therapy are fatigue, dry mouth, cataracts, permanent hair loss, problems with memory, infertility, issues with thyroid or adrenal glands, sensitive skin when exposed to the sun, and developing secondary cancers. This section will focus on hair loss, infertility, dry mouth, and lung problems.

Hair loss: Only the part of the body under radiation is subject to hair loss. Losing hair on your leg because of radiation doesn't cause head hair to disappear. The damage will depend on factors like the total dose given and the size of the area that was a target for radiation. Hair loss can also occur in the area where the radiation beam exits the body. Like chemotherapy, radiation destroys healthy cells in its path. It damages those cells that grow at fast rates, including hair cells causing loss or thinning of hair.

Each patient situation concerning hair loss is unique and depends on the amount of radiation received. If the patient receives high doses of radiation, then hair loss may be permanent. On the contrary, if low doses are received, hair loss could be temporary. Sometimes, even small doses of radiation can lead to permanent hair loss. When the hair grows back, if it does, it won't change color, but changes in texture may be noticeable.

Hair loss could be a substantial problem for some people, particularly those who care about their looks or have a job that requires glamour as a basis such as modeling. There are no right or wrong responses to losing your hair. Each person reacts to the situation in their way and what makes them comfortable. For those who are a little more sensitive to the loss of hair and the *possibility* of losing their hair is high, try to shave your head before treatment to get the feel before the actual hair loss occurs. After therapy, protect your head with a hat to keep away the sunlight. Try not to use a hair dryer, hot rollers, or curling irons and avoid bleaching your hair or changing the color since the chemical can make your hair fall out. A visit to an experienced hairstylist can make your life easier.

Infertility: The use of radiation in women can kill cancer cells, but it can also cause damage to the woman's ovaries. High doses always inflict some damage; here, they destroy some or all the eggs in the ovaries, leading to infertility and early menopause. Infertility can result from radiation therapy depending on the area treated. The inability to have children after receiving radiation can be temporary or permanent. Likewise, radiation directed at the brain can affect the pituitary gland, which controls the hormonal agents necessary to produce eggs and sperm. If radiation targets the abdominal area—for example, pelvis and reproductive organs—it can impact the fertility of females and men but in different ways.

The effect of radiation on men can be substantial if the area near the testicles is targeted. It may reduce sperm production, resulting in a dry orgasm, which is when you feel the sensation of an orgasm but ejaculates little or no semen. Production of semen often is restored after a few months, but for some men, the effect is permanent and causes infertility. Erection could also be an issue after receiving radiation therapy because of nerve damage and the severity of the side effects depends on how much radiation you have received. According to the Mayo Clinic, radiation may also damage nerves in your pelvic area, block blood flow to your penis, or decrease the level of testosterone in your body, and may reduce the amount of semen you ejaculate. The medical community has performed research on repairing the damage and restoring erectile dysfunction caused by radiation, but this is still in their experimental stage.

Dry mouth: Dry mouth is also called xerostomia. Along with chemotherapy, radiation therapy can cause dry mouth by damaging the salivary glands. Radiation to the head, face, or neck may also cause dry mouth. It's a temporary problem that lasts between two to eight weeks. Damaging the salivary glands stops them from making the saliva necessary to keep the mouth moist, and your ability to chew, taste, and swallow requires spit to accomplish the job.

Dry-mouth relief is possible through medicines and saliva substitutes. However, there are various things you can do to heal your dry mouth and feel comfortable. Taking care of your teeth through regular visits to the dentist and frequent brushing and flossing will help with the effect after receiving radiation. Drink sips of water to make up for the lost moisture and avoid mouthwashes that contain alcohol. Use a humidifier with cool mist at night while you sleep. Avoid caffeine and acidic sodas; eat soft, moist foods; and avoid hard foods and those that burn your mouth.

Lung problems: Complications with lungs can happen when the doctor directs radiation at the chest, resulting in lung damage. You may experience shortness of breath, wheezing, fever, dry cough, congestion, and exhaustion, where oxygen therapy may be required if you have trouble breathing. Doctors give oxygen through nasal prongs or a mask that fits over your mouth and nose. Sometimes, you may get oxygen through a ventilator.

Along with the doctor's recommendations, the most important thing to do is to avoid smoking and secondhand smoking. Your physician can prescribe medications to help you unwind when it's tough to breathe, to ease and treat discomfort. Taking steroid pills to help with lung problems can disrupt the way the body uses certain nutrients, including calcium, potassium, sodium, and protein. Here, it's essential to eat a well-balanced diet recommended by your nutritional expert. A healthy diet plan comprised of foods from each food group can make up for some impacts of steroid treatment.

RECURRENCE

Cancer recurrence is most feared among cancer patients, especially those who are cancer-free—sometimes measured in months or even years after finishing the treatment when recurrence can happen. When cancer could not be detected, another one may appear. This is called recurrence, and it's related to your primary cancer.

Recurrence might resurface in the same place that your primary cancer started, or it might occur in a different part of your body. Naming the new cancer is based on the name of the original one even if it has invaded other parts of the body. For example, if you had a prostate cancer that, after some time, spreads to the bones, then a new tumor will be named after the first cancer, a prostate cancer, and will be treated like prostate cancer. Tests will be done to find out similarities and differences. Predicting when and if cancer will come back isn't possible, but it's harder to treat it, and it's more likely to resurface if it's a fast-growing or a more aggressive (advanced) cancer that had spread to other parts of the body. Although predicting recurrence is hard to do, but your doctor will give you an idea about the probability of recurrence, depending on your situation.

There are a few different cancer recurrence types:

- o Local recurrence is when cancer has come back in the same place.

- Regional recurrence means that cancer has come back in the lymph nodes near the area it first started.
- Distant recurrence implies cancer has come back in another part of the body, some distance from where it began (the lungs, bone, brain, or liver).

Although the recurrent cancer is related to your first primary cancer, as opposed to second cancer unrelated to the primary one, the concept of reemergence or recurrence differs from progression. It's difficult to tell the difference between the two phenomena. Progression is when cancer gets worse. For example, if cancer comes back after a few months, how do you know if it's recurrence or progression? Chances are this is no recurrence. This issue could arise if, after surgery, a few tiny clusters of cancerous cells were left behind because of the difficulty of detecting them through scans. These cells develop and come back to form cancer again. Another possibility is when cancer or some of the remaining cells become resistant to chemotherapy. Those leftover cells can grow again to develop cancer, and it usually happens when it's advanced and very aggressive. There's no standard length of time to decide if it's a recurrence or progression; often, when the return time is short, it means that the situation is dangerous. However, most doctors consider recurrence to be cancer that comes back after you've had no signs for at least a year.

As the situation with many cancers, there are a few things you can do to slow their growth or even stop their progression to a certain degree, including eating right, exercising, a few changes in lifestyle, and seeing your doctor regularly. A critical item in the list is to learn how to abide by your follow-up care plan and miss no routine testing. However, even if you do everything right, cancer still might come back.

Despite what your doctor says after you complete your treatment, there's always a chance that cancer may come back. Even if your doctor says that your cancer is gone or that he removed it, there's no guarantee it won't come back. Recurrence of cancer has common signs. There are only a few significant symptoms that could mean serious problems for your type of cancer. Your doctor should make you aware of these symptoms if they exist in your case.

Talk to your doctor if you have any of the signs listed in chapter 2. Those signs could be unrelated to cancer but could be because of other illnesses, such as the flu, colds, infections, heart problems, arthritis, and so on. Besides the common cancer signs and symptoms covered in chapter 2 under the abbreviations CAUTION, watch for weight loss, unusual pain unrelated to an injury that doesn't go away, easy bleeding and bruising, chills, fevers, blood in the stool or urine, shortness of breath, or anything you think it's abnormal.[R49]

DEVELOPING SECOND CANCERS

The development of second cancers differs from recurrence. Second cancers (unrelated to the first one) aren't common, but they occur. If tests show a new tumor is of a different type than the first primary cancer, then you would have two kinds or two primary cancers. These two kinds of cancer would have started in different types of cells and will look different under the microscope, which is much rarer than cancer recurrence. You can be at a higher risk of getting second cancers than a nonpatient. The initial cancer treatment (radiation therapy and chemotherapy) that you have received for your cancer can sometimes cause new cancer to appear many years after you have finished treatment. When this occurs, it's known as a second primary cancer.[R50]

The journey has been long and filled with turbulence. Despite the details, you should be proud of arriving at this point and congratulations on such a spectacular accomplishment. Now is the perfect time to examine and assess your life and apply what you will learn to strengthen your progress.

CHAPTER FOURTEEN

EVALUATE YOUR LIFE

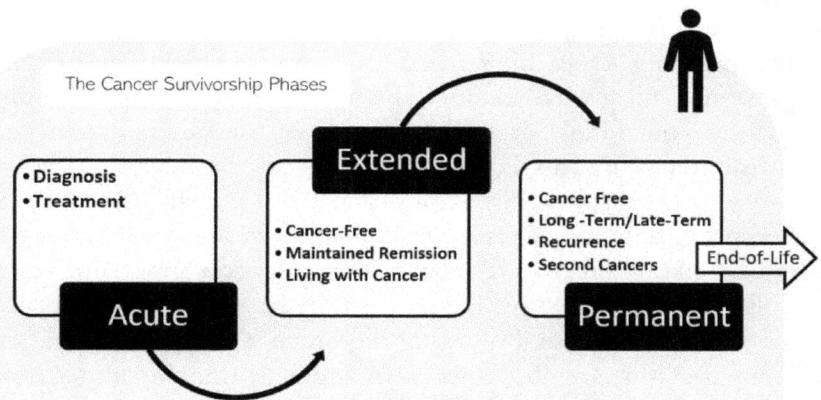

It's time to evaluate your life

You're in the permanent phase. You're cancer-free, may have had second cancer or cancer recurrence, or you're merely managing your cancer as a chronic illness. Despite your condition, you must move forward and continue to administer your current health situation. Implementing what you have learned in the past can help you evaluate your life to either sustain current health or improve your prognosis. If you're nearing the end of life, skip to chapter 15 to learn about the various ways to make the final months, weeks, or days as easy as possible for you and your loved ones.

Some people call this era of the patient's journey the "after-cancer" season. I'm not eager to accept this term because it doesn't convey an accurate description of the individual's position on the cancer continuum. The term *after cancer* can mean after diagnosis, irrespective of the outcomes, and the stage of the disease. If you're reading this chapter because you need information depicting your place in your cancer journey in the permanent survivorship phase, then you're living a "new normal." What's important here is that you're still alive where enjoyment and excellent quality of life await you. This period of your journey brings many questions about the pursuit of life's purpose and discovering its meaning.

Your life purpose changed with cancer, but your feelings bring you meaning. Does life's meaning comprise everything within your passion? Or is it what you love and what brings you happiness and joy, such as your family or a job? Outside of the cancer experience, our surroundings draw us to events like a tragedy, birth, or an occasion that forced us to shape our lives. But cancer is personal and will change us because, often, it catalyzes a modification in our lives. Serious health issues like cancer will draw on resources you might never oblige yourself to use before—strength, resilience, and perhaps emotions you dislike. Following the cancer experience, it's rational to compare the past with the present and start thinking about how you want to live going forward. Sometimes, we feel enthusiastic and rewarded about future changes, and other times, we're overwhelmed and discouraged.

Is there a perfect way of identifying a life's purpose? How do we know we're reaching what we desire in life? Cancer patients have opposing views about life's purpose and meaning; some say beating cancer itself is their life purpose. Others say cancer has given them a new purpose in life, pushing them to carry out a more fulfilling life using all resources available to them. Despite opposing views, they should look at it as a fluid construct that evolves in time, which has various markers we assess against as we need to, which enables us to recognize where on a scale we are. So I might sense that a three-month sabbatical away from home is a time when I find significance and function in my life. I'm high on the scale, but my return is rocky and uncertain. I step down one degree, but I take up running as a pastime, which I enjoy. Then I am at a higher grade, creating new friends, making me climb upward again.

WHAT BRINGS US MEANING?

It's what motivates you to become happy, including spending time with family, going to work, traveling, and so on. It differs for people. What might seem small but satisfactory for some may not feel the same for others. Now is the perfect moment to look for your purpose. Understanding your values makes you focus your time on activities, projects, or living overall in a way that meets those values.

Cancer will change you despite your weaknesses and strengths. It will teach you to be content with the unknown, but you'll also learn how to accept your surroundings and test things out—ideas, projects, hobbies, even whole lifestyles—to assess how right you feel. Sometimes you don't have to change to learn to adjust; simple changes may accomplish the job. Accepting threats and vulnerabilities may include testing brand-new things out in your life, such as something you need to get used to—as if you needed to feel more susceptible. However, this time, it can be within your control and through the choices you make. So ask yourself what makes you happy? What's the one thing you wanted to accomplish in life but could not because of surprises? Can you work on it now? Can you imagine a happy period of your life that you can replicate? Think positive and work hard at getting what you desire.

Upon reading hundreds of stories portraying the lives of cancer survivors and mentoring a similar number of patients through their journeys, I realized that they all shared a common denominator, the search for a new meaning for life. To them, cancer and death go hand in hand. Many of them worked hard at reevaluating the meaning of life and started appreciating the simple things in life. Some of them told me they were being reborn again as infants and had to review their lives to serve as mentors to others new to this disease.

Evaluation of your new life means you must learn to adapt to changing circumstances that occur daily. Pay attention to everything that makes up your life, and prioritize to adjust to the new environment. Your sense of normalcy is evolving, but you'll find peace within yourself and accept life and the "new normal." As time goes on, you feel much better, gain strength, and feel more like yourself.

When you first heard of your diagnosis, your perception of time changed, and you had to put a limitation on the length of your life. Through the process, you tried to rush almost everything to squeeze as much as you can with the time limit you had set for yourself. You become impatient, get angry with little things, become more sensitive, and grow frustrated. However, all this will happen while you're trying to regain your sense of normalcy again. You appreciate the time you have and take advantage of every single minute of the day. Your life gets saturated with good as opposed to evil. You have a greater sense of support and compassion, ease of forgiveness, and your inner strength will increase, and you think of your everyday life much differently. The unpredictability of your future will alter your thought processes about your top priorities, profession, family, and good friends.

No one understands what you're going through or what your life feels like dealing with cancer. It's natural for people around you not to understand the reality of your situation since they have never experienced the same. They might think the cancer experience stops when treatment ends. Family and friends want to see you recovered and distress-free, and some of them might act differently around you. Explain to them what's happening and let them know that you seek their support while you adapt to changes.

Cancer affects people in various ways. Remember the story of my friend Mark at the doctor's office? Mark received the news of his cancer diagnosis with ease. At least, that's what his facial expressions at that moment revealed. I accompanied Mark for the next ten months after his initial diagnosis until his death. During that period of his sickness, he acted like he always did, calm and confident. Mark started thinking about doing all the simple things he wanted to do but either ignored or procrastinated. But he never rushed to do them because he never imagined his life could expire so quickly. He was positive throughout his cancer journey and started doing more than what he usually did. He even started exercising and eating healthy foods, stuff he never did before his diagnosis.

Some of my patients refuse to change their lives to adapt to the new environment; they are happy with the past and want to continue with their routines. My advice to them is to do whatever pleases them without exertion. I tell them to think about what they intend to do and do it; to focus on essentials and seek activities such as meditations, yoga, and rest; and to always prepare themselves for mixed reactions from family and friends. If people don't know how to react, try not to get upset. Some people avoid contact because cancer brings up painful emotions. They are dealing with it in their own way.[R51]

FINDING THE "NEW NORMAL"

Many people see a positive side to having cancer; it enables them to discover their inner strength and revise their outlook on life. Others may find new delightful avenues concerning relationships and sources of support. Your life priorities change. You value people more and have better relationships with spouse and family. You find excitement in traveling and improve the way you look at your job or career. And you may change your lifestyle into a better one. It's a new chapter in a new life with hopes, happiness, and fewer worries.

It's time to cope with all that you've experienced. Your coping ability and strategies differ from everyone else's. You must think about what the experience did to your family, friends, job, and your relationships. The financial matter may stress you, and your anxiety is high again. Start with the following to help you progress.

- **Think about the periods of your diagnosis and treatment.** Analyze the feelings you had in both situations; what worried you the most during those periods? Take a moment to reflect on the past and use it as a tool to look forward to your future.
- **Stop thinking you're alone.** Your health-care team members will still help you, and although it may seem like they aren't always there compared to the past, they started to become like family members. But suddenly, they are busy with someone else; you aren't the main star anymore—a sad event that can make you feel lonely and abandoned. The same is true for family members and close friends; they were always there for you; now, they went on with their lives; this can only add to your feelings of loneliness and frustration. Understand that all those people are still there, but they have their own lives to run.
- **Don't hide your feelings**. People around you who never had cancer will never know how you feel. Don't consider it as negligence on their part; they don't know. If their action affects

you, tell them how you feel on the inside and that you're trying to recover and seek support from your surroundings.
- **Don't rush for a change.** Also, accept the reality of your health and work toward gaining that spot again. Allow yourself time to adjust. The time factor is essential; returning to normal health takes time and effort and depends on the severity of your cancer.
- **Don't worry about what people think.** Never try to impress anyone just because you want to appear normal to them. Act like yourself, focus on the ones you care about, let them know about the new you. If you believe that you should be thankful, then that's okay, but it's also okay to feel angry, frustrated, depressed, or whatever, but again, don't change for anyone except for yourself.
- **Change essential priorities.** There may be times when you have to think about changing your most critical priorities, such as your work situation. Work is vital since it provides you with a source of income, and it's the one thing that takes the most out of your time and energy. Changing priorities concerning work will be the most challenging decision. The effects of cancer and treatment may motivate or deter you from returning or staying at work.
- **Stay hopeful.** Take the time to enjoy yourself with family and friends—times filled with happiness and meaning. Keep doing what you love, and don't let this beast stop you from enjoying your life. And always hope for the best. Nobody knows when the end will happen.

But how do you accomplish all that? It's easier said than done, but there are a few things you can do to change some priorities that may impact your decisions:

- The time factor is the one element that allows you to accomplish essential tasks. Since your job is the most time-consuming issue, you think about spending part or all that time with family and loved ones instead of being at work. You may think being at work takes time away from being with loved ones. Weigh the benefits and risks of working less at your job before you plan to adjust your work situation.

- The desire to live mindfully. Eagerness may include being more aware of living in the moment at home and work—this area takes practice and compassion. It's fine to put yourself first, and it's ok to embrace a new perspective on life without ignoring emotional struggles as they arise.
- To look at the positive outcomes of cancer. Yes, there are positive outcomes of this dreadful disease. Cancer is an event in your life that will produce negative and positive consequences. By now, it's clear how cancer impacted your life. Some changes in your life are apparent early on; others may be subtle and take a while to develop. Some changes might provide themselves as alternatives—options that you might reject or accept. Counting the ways life will be better during this period of your journey is something positive.
- Start thinking about how to improve and enjoy your life each day. Your days become filled with quality time enjoyed by you and your family, friends, and coworkers. Whenever you do something new like an adventure or plan a dream trip, you'll make sure that every minute counts, and you'll do your best to enjoy it with all you've got.
- You may be one of the fortunate patients who will hear the doctor say that your cancer may be gone; he might even say that your cancer may be gone forever. Imagine how ecstatic you'll be.
- It's a happy day when your treatment ends. You feel you're born again, no more scheduled appointments with your doctor (well, maybe a few), no more hospitals, and no more pain. Now you can plan your days to do some other things you love instead of expecting to get up early in the morning to receive chemotherapy or other forms of torture. You're free to go to the gym, spa, swim, volunteer, and whatever pleases you and fulfills your days with joy.
- Your fear recedes, and you aren't afraid anymore. Each passing day, your fear dissipates, and the more you try to enjoy yourself, the more fear disappears until you go back to normal again, a life with no doubt. In years to come—and we have this on good authority from long-time survivors—you may even forget that you have cancer unless reminded of its presence. Envision that!

- You'll be adventurous, no fear. Your hair grew back, no drugs. You have a sense of daring, a wild side. You want to travel and explore and enjoy every minute.
- You become stronger in every sense. You have been through hell and back; all this strengthened you, and you became more experienced. You have passed the difficult test, and you survived. It's quite an accomplishment to survive cancer.
- Everything around you, including people, becomes more meaningful. Your relationships with people improve; you realize there's no sense in having issues with people.
- You forgive more now, and you don't hold grudges because it isn't worth the anger and the worry, only wisdom and compassion toward others; hence, you gain importance with others. Being grateful to be alive doesn't imply accepting whatever others throw at you, and it doesn't prevent sticking up for yourself when others upset you.
- Support for others grows naturally. You want to help anyone who needs help and reduce their pain. You speak the language of the disease now, and you'll want to use the knowledge gained on those who are still suffering.
- One minute, you look in the mirror and choose not to wear your wig, and the next, you visit your hairstylist to get a haircut.
- Time flies; however, after cancer, you treasure the time you have and make the most of it.

Don't expect to go back to normal unless you work on executing the points outlined above and take care of the side effects that you may be experiencing. If you succeed, then you're on your way back to normal or close to it.[R5]

MOVING FORWARD

The only way to stay healthy is to have a positive outlook. Staying positive and having the right attitude help you focus so you can take care of the many details lying ahead. Learn how to live with uncertainty about recurrence and the precautions you should undertake to minimize the chances. These thoughts may keep you up at night, and that's normal. This uncertainty may stay with you for years after treatment. Every follow-up visit, the anniversary of the diagnosis and treatment, and other events are reminders, or if anyone else gets cancer, it's still a reminder, or worse yet, if someone you know has a recurrence. Illness of a family member having symptoms similar to yours when your disease appeared or the death of someone because of cancer can trigger these feelings of uncertainty. You must erase all obstacles, including negative thinking, to enable you to move forward. The following short list contains a few tips to help you attain the best outcomes of your continued journey:

- Learn about your surroundings, people, health-care personnel, resources, and what available services and support systems can do for you. You'll get a touch of gratification in learning of such help.
- Let go, or manage, the fear you may have because of your thoughts about recurrence. Your cancer may never come back.
- Know your present health and know that some cancer treatments may induce health issues later on. Ask your cancer-care team if your health-and-wellness concerns are only brief or whether they are long-term. Ask for a piece of advice on how to learn about them and what to do if you notice them.
- Managing your health-care records can be a complicated endeavor, particularly if you're juggling information from various medical providers and other sources, such as pharmacies and insurance companies. However, saving copies of your records and knowing how to find them is essential to improving the high quality of care you receive, especially if you change doctors. You need copies of the pathology reports, imaging tests results, surgery (if any), all biopsies' reports, and records of your hospital stay. Include the dates and types of treatments you have received. Gather as much information as possible about your health-care team members, including all the doctors you have seen since your diagnosis day.
- Insurance coverage is vital to help pay the high cancer costs. Make sure you keep paying the premium on your insurance to keep it active. Insurance companies won't hesitate to end your coverage if you stop paying your bills on time. You might have difficulties paying for your insurance since you may have had to stop work for a while or even have changed jobs. Finances

can be hard at these difficult times, so do what you must do to keep your insurance active. If you're sixty-five or older, you can get Medicare. It's difficult to get medical insurance if cancer comes back. Insurance rates can be high in your situation, but cancer treatment and care cost way more.

- o As part of the routine follow-up visits, your doctor may request additional medical testing to ensure that cancer has not returned. Such tests may include blood tests and imaging scans. Depending on your cancer, the doctors may request specific exams. For example, if you have prostate cancer, you may have to take prostate-specific antigen (PSA) blood tests every six months for the first five years. Testing is often done at least annually after that. Seeing your doctor and the health-care team according to your routine checkup schedule will help to monitor your situation and detect a recurrence, if any, early. Here your cancer team will watch you to ensure that there are no signs of cancer recurrence.
- o At some point, you may seek a new doctor or health-care facility. It's imperative to present them with the details of your diagnosis and treatment. One of the best means to help your provider get precise information is to provide them with copies of your clinical records. It's challenging to get clinical documents that are greater than a few years old, so it's best if you can collect this information throughout your therapy. If you aren't sure where to start, ask your cancer-care team how to get your medical reports.[R53]

You're the pilot of this long, turbulent journey, and no one is better able than you to reach safe ground when it's your life you're piloting. By now, you know that attaining your goals is only possible with perseverance and determination strengthened by knowledge. You can live the healthy life you always dreamed of, even after facing all the obstacles cancer threw at you. But some cancer patients will reach a point in their journey when they must transition into the end-of-life period. If you're one of those patients, then proceed to the next chapter to learn about ways to transition less painfully for you and your loved ones. I have included the next chapter, "Restate Your Priorities,' as part of the survivorship strategy since you're still called a *survivor* until the moment you die. This chapter is particularly beneficial for caregivers and family members who are taking care of their beloved patient during the end of life period.

CHAPTER FIFTEEN

RESTATE YOUR PRIORITIES

END-OF-LIFE

You've reached the end of the road; perhaps you stopped treatment since you've concluded that your situation is worsening or therapy is ineffective anymore. Your decision to stop treatment also may have been because you developed a second aggressive cancer, or your cancer came back with a vengeance. I doubt if any choice of words would diminish your anguish, but I can at least try to comfort you with my past experience with cancer patients who had similar experiences. In your final days or weeks, there are a few things you can undertake to make the transitional period less agonizing on you and those close to your heart.

When your body stops responding to treatment, and your doctor determines that treatment should end, or when you stop treatment for any other reasons, you might have a few months, perhaps a few weeks, even days before death occurs. Your fundamental ignorance of such an appalling experience clears the path to immense feelings of being alone and afraid. You realize that cancer isn't going away, and the time left is limited. During the final days, the emphasis of health care, in the form of palliative or hospice care, will be on improving your quality of life.

This chapter explores emotions and physical signals in the last two to three months of your life and values the importance of communication with family members, close friends, and the health-care team. Information in this chapter is also beneficial for loved ones and caregivers who are accompanying you during this difficult time.

EMOTIONS DURING THE FINAL DAYS

Death is an event beyond our comprehension, and we know all that is living will vanish; only memories remain. The repercussion of death is rather clear: a life—with all that word implies—ends.

Awareness that you're departing this life can provoke overwhelming sensations of fear and solitude. Fear of the unknown ahead, both the way of dying and the fear of the mystification after death, can produce guilt, stress, and anxiety as you look back at your life. Death delivers an end to a conflict with others, some of whom you're associated with, although detached. The time comes to "clean up" the life, pulling in the loose ends to fashion a clean break. Despite the ravages of the illness and its treatments, you can die healthy in mind and spirit. In dying, you can bring life back, in the sense that you define and make personal relationships with others and with the world explicit.

Please understand that during the final days, a plethora of emotional elements seems to find its place inside your circle of caregivers, family, and friends. Almost everyone involved experiences enduring episodes of confusion, sorrow, despair, and empathy. Often, when your caregivers and family members know that what you may experience toward the end-of-life period will give them the strength to better care for you, they will help themselves survive these hard times.

During the end-of-life period, something enhances your emotions to their highest levels. Some of these emotions are anger, guilt, regret, grieve, anxiety, depression, feeling alone, and fear of the unknown. You'll try to seek any information that will give meaning to what's happening.

Fear is a reasonable response to believing death is near, and its impact on you varies with different individuals. Identifying what part of death is triggering this fear can be helpful. Some people are frightened of the unknown; some are afraid of dying alone or troubled about the pain during the moment of death and what comes after death. Knowing about the specific reasons triggering fear may help you manage the final days with less anguish. If being alone is frightening, share it with loved ones so they can be beside you.

Anger is a normal reaction to dying and knowing that departure from life is imminent. It's also a common reaction caused by feeling embarrassed after an emotional outburst. It's a strong emotion, a powerful release of frustration. You might scream to relieve annoyance and ask questions like "Why me?" or "What have I done to deserve this?" You may show this expression in the form of yelling, sarcasm, hostility, or display of aggression. Anger can give rise to guilt since the release of anger and frustration can offend or push away loved ones and friends when you need them most. Identify what you experience as angry behaviors and determine the cause to ease your anger toward people around you.

Guilt and regret are among the many emotions you'll feel during the final days of life. Guilt and regret develop when you think you're a burden on family members and for leaving loved ones behind, like children. You may regret things you've done either to induce cancer or other stuff you wish you could have done and hope you can go back and change the past.

Grief is an intense feeling, likely to be very pronounced in the last few months. It may be the most remarkable effect, besides fear—no more plans, no more spending time with loved ones, no more vacations, and no more future. Everything comes to a halt. You may have lost many things already, such as the strength to accomplish simple tasks or walk around like you used to, or interest in many things you used to do, such as eating your favorite food or getting up whenever you desire to go for a small run. You may feel isolated from your friends and can't handle that you'll leave them. Many physical and emotional losses happen just before death itself. Those you love are grieving also, knowing that you won't be around anymore. How can you and your loved ones discover significance in what's taking place? Try to talk with your loved ones about the sorrow and loss of dreams you're all experiencing. Having the ability to rise above the pain and connect to something higher than oneself may assist you and your loved ones to heal after you're gone.

Anxiety and depression are like anything else that is substantial during this period. You feel it in your guts. Even healthy individuals become anxious and depressed about many things in life, including small and silly events. Anxiety and depression are maximal during this agonizing time; symptoms could include a nervous stomach, shaky feelings all over, being short-tempered, a sense of dread or worry, or fear of the unknown. Helplessness, desperation, and feeling useless may accompany you, sometimes until the end. Anxiety and depression can increase your fear of death, which must be treated with medications and perhaps counseling. Prescribed medications might be necessary to lessen the effects on you and stop them from serving as an obstacle to a harmonious atmosphere during this challenging time.

Feeling alone is a renowned perception of nearing death, and therefore, mental isolation may emerge, you might experience loneliness even if people are present. Many of my patients told me they were feeling isolated when people were filling the room, also when their spouses and their young children are present. Feeling alone occurs because of the accumulation of all the unfavorable emotional elements accompanying you during the period of dying. The mind is occupied trying to repair negativity in every way, causing you to become isolated from the world around you. Discuss your loneliness with those closest to you and ask them to stay around and keep you occupied with positive thoughts.

Seeking meaning may have been lost during the end-of-life period. Almost everyone wants to feel that life has a purpose and there is a reason for being on earth. Thoughts of gaining answers about life's meaning and purpose intensify during the period of dying. Death means that whatever goal you think you had for a living will end soon, and to reach what you think you were living for is impossible. You become heartbroken, knowing you can't proceed with the life purpose you set for yourself. [R54]

SIGNS THE END IS NEAR

Each person's journey to the end-of-life is unique; for some people, death can occur fast, whereas, for others, the decline is gradual.

Knowing some signs that emerge when the end is nearing prepares you for many unknowns. These signs help both you and your caregivers to manage this difficult period to reduce the substantial trauma that will affect everyone involved. Some changes you may expect when the body stops working are a normal part of dying, and every patient will experience all the signs with varying intensity depending on many elements, including the age of the patient. Children and teens have a similar process, although it can be harder to predict since they often stay active and continue to ask a lot of tough-to-answer questions. Death of a child can inflict a damaging effect on caregivers and family members, sometimes irreversible. This event might require serious psychological counseling for some family members to help with coping.

One to three months before death, the patient will sleep and doze more, eating and drinking habits change, avoid and detest people, speak less, and feel lonely. The confusion about the situation makes the signs of death for younger people more substantial, depending on the severity of their cancers. They share most of the warning signals with adults except walking more.

One to two weeks before death, the patient will feel exhausted all the time. They could develop some different sleep-wake patterns, changes in appetite, fewer and smaller bowel movements, less pee, more pain, changes in breathing, and variations in blood pressure and heart rate. Body temperature fluctuates and may leave their skin cold, warm, moist, or pale. The patient experiences congested breathing from fluid buildup in the throat's back. Also, confusion or what looks like being in a daze emerges as a glaring sign. Breathing often isn't painful and can be managed. Treating pain is possible. However, loved ones may have a hard time taking medicine by mouth. Hallucination and vision problems are apparent during this period.

Within the last few days, also called the "active-dying" phase, blood pressure drops, the patient is in a coma or semicoma. The patient refuses food or drinks, stops peeing or having bowel movements. Grimacing, groaning, or scowling from pain becomes apparent, and you may see tears or eyes glaze over. Pulse is hard to feel, the heartbeat is irregular and hard to hear, and body temperature level drops. The skin on knees, feet, and hands turns a mottled bluish-purple (in the last twenty-four hours). Breathing is disrupted by gasping and slows until it stops. Your loved one might drift in and out if they're not already unconscious. They can still feel and hear.

In the last few hours, the patient becomes restless and confused. Hallucination becomes so upsetting they may cry out, strike out, or try to climb out of bed. Calming can be accomplished through the use of relaxing music. Sometimes, medication helps.

Although learning about the signs can be helpful when knowing when to start preparing, predicting "active dying" can be a challenge since the patient may not exhibit all the initial signals of dying. Sometimes the patient knows the end is very near, and he or she may make it known. Often the patient's position will become rigid, showing that the time of death has approached.

THE IMPORTANCE OF COMMUNICATION

Planning for the remaining time of your life demands effective communication with various people, including your health-care team members. Getting answers to all your questions gives you a sense of control over what's coming. Although the health-care team may do nothing anymore, they can help you plan so you won't feel alone and confused. Every little piece of information helps, so you must try to be open and honest with them. It helps your situation a lot if you can establish channels of communication with your partners, family members, friends, and with your spiritual or religious counselors if you have any.

Communicate with your partner. Your partner is the individual you shared many difficulties with, so there must be a lot to debate. Focus on good times instead of the bad. Remember that emotions are high for both of you, depending on your partner and the life you've shared with this person. Some people might pull away if they can't handle the circumstance, and that could be very painful for you. Even their presence could be painful if you shared memories.

Knowing you'll leave them, if there is an expected burden on them after you leave, will make it harder to deal with the situation. Sometimes partners attempt to safeguard each other from the pain they're both going through; however, when this transpires, they may sacrifice honesty. Walls of uneasiness will divide both partners, making you avoid certain topics, and relationships can become strained and uncomfortable. Try to accept what the other person is saying without arguing or denouncing each other, and don't fix the feelings. Pronounce your love and care for each other and leave the bad times in the past to create a chance to reverse past wrongs to become a source of comfort. However, having cancer doesn't mean you won't get frustrated and mad at each other. Try to bring warmth into the spotlight and let minor arguments go. Concentrate on the great times and happy memories, and give each other alone time. When people are dying, they may want to be alone sometimes to gather their thoughts.

What happens to sex and intimacy? At this point in the disease, it's difficult to deal with sex and intimacy, and you may be exhausted, in some pain, or just not interested in sex. However, you can keep physical contact in your relationship and share intimacy. Speaking about it resolves most of the problems. Establish that your partner understands that you want physical closeness and affection. Touching, hugging, and holding hands may feel more intimate than other forms of physical contact.

Communicate with your family. Cancer is a family illness, and each member of the family will have their share of suffering. Excellent communication with family members reduces the strain on everyone involved. Let them know you're open to a discussion about anything and the source of their feelings and talk about it. Be truthful about your emotional and physical pain. Speak to them about the future without you and how to deal with it and what to do and prepare themselves during the final days and hours. Tell them about your plans and get their input, but be honest and careful about the choice of words. Talking to the younger generation should take on a different format. Children can pick up changes or tension in the household and understand when something is wrong. Sometimes what they picture is far worse than anything you tell them.

Communicate with your friends. Not all your friends react the same way to dying. Some friends will meet your expectations and behave in the same way you expected. They will be excellent listeners and become available and around you for the duration of the process. Some others will feel uncomfortable; they may appear overwhelmed and don't understand what to say. They won't know how to operate around you and may seem to have a tough time being "normal." In certain situations, minor discomfort may accompany those who are beside you, when that happens, try to talk to them about their troubles and make them feel a bit at ease. If they're prepared to do that, discuss that you're the same individual, and you would like to invest some of your remaining time with them. Strive to recognize what you're going through may trigger your loved ones to think about the reality they, too, will die. Considering that this isn't a pleasurable thing, some people may avoid associating with you.

Communicate with religious counselors. According to leading religions, death is a part of life; it's a natural end of the gift of life, a transition to another, yet unknown, existence. Religion can be a cause of strength for believing patients and their loved ones. Some patients transitioning into the end-of-life period will even resort to prayer, although they may never have had religious faith or accepted a higher power. Others aren't concerned or attached to any religious systems or beliefs and may not have the urge to turn to religion. During this challenging time, many people, including the patient, may have tough questions about illness and life. Some of those questions may seem irrational, but religion can answer most. Talking to a spiritual or religious counselor may help you and your loved ones find comfort and contentment. The counselor may encourage religious practices, such as forgiveness, confession, or praying; they can be assuring and bring you a sense of peace. Interested patients should resort to a minister, imam, priest, rabbi, another clergy member, or a skilled pastoral therapist to help determine the spiritual requirements and find spiritual support.

UNFINISHED BUSINESS

It's imperative for you and your close family members to start a discussion concerning various delicate issues once treatment stops. Examples include the acceptance or rejection of a feeding tube or pain medication. Also, you might find that some individuals won't accept your choice to cease cancer treatment. Even if they don't agree or comprehend, you still need to follow your sense of what's right for you. If you've explored all the options leading to halting treatment, your family and friends will more than likely support you. Keep in mind that no decision is permanent; you can always alter your account. Still, it's your decision, and you should be comfortable with it. You might wish to share the reasons for your choice so they can better understand the circumstances leading to such a decision. Making your medical team and your close family members part of the decision-making process will help the situation in the most efficient way possible. You may prefer to concentrate on the quality of life and spare yourself from the adverse effects of cancer treatment, although it's important to know your doctor can always deal with any side effects.

It isn't the act of dying, but it's the quality that is of concern at the end of life. Most people who come to accept death as a natural and fundamental part of life don't want to lengthen the process when it doesn't change the outcome, however, considering a good death isn't something most people do. Some patients wish to remain at home and take advantage of hospice care. Others may go to an assisted-living center, an assisted-living home, or an inpatient hospice program. Some remain in the health-care facility and desire any treatment offered to prolong their life if possible, no matter what their condition might be. Once again, it would be best if you made the choices you feel are best for you, your family, and your circumstances.

Any cancer care intends to allow you to take advantage of the best support to have a good quality of life. At this moment, it's imperative to prepare for how you'll die, not just how you'll live in the next few months.

Advance directives: These are legal documents prepared by an attorney or any other legal personality for eliminating inevitable disagreements about the patient's health care toward the end-of-life period. These are legal documents (for example, a power of attorney and a will) that are crucial in eliminating disputes between loved ones should a disagreement occur. Advance directives reveal your wishes for health-care members if you cannot make your intentions known because of severe impairment. In those documents, you can name what person you wish to make decisions for you. Understand that it's always your right to accept or decline any health care, including cancer treatment. The patient must consider crucial legal documentation during the end-of-life period, and I always emphasized focusing on this matter when the end was near, usually in the last two to three months before dying.

Without a directive, you're leaving the decisions about your health care to others, and you may not get the health care you want, or you may get the health care you don't wish to receive; it's that simple. Others can decide for you when you can't decide yourself. If you have made your wishes known earlier, you don't need advance directives concerning the health-care segment of your end-of-life journey. Advance directives are only designated to discuss health-care choices and may not go against the doctor's morals or the intention to break the facility's rules or health-care standards.

A clear example of advance directives could be in the form of a living will, such as stating your wishes about a specific health treatment at the end of life. To execute a living will, you must have a life-ending illness or be unconscious for the rest of your life. It could be in the form of a durable power of attorney to name the person who will be a decision-maker concerning your health care, such as in the case of a treatment you don't wish to receive.

Inside the document, you can state if you wish to stay on the machines necessary to sustain your life including CPR, chest compression, breathing devices, nutrition and fluids, others that do the job of a kidney, or certain types of medicines. Included also in the document, you could state whether you want comfort care, a treatment that would make you more comfortable, such as pain medications. You can enclose a DNR (do not resuscitate) demand, such as restarting your heart or lungs in case they stop working. In the advance directive, you could add whether you want to stay at home or live in a hospital for the specified period. Other parts of the document may include organ donation in case you wish to donate some of your organs upon death.

Consult with your attorney about the procedure and give copies to the people who will decide for you. Keep a copy in your wallet and leave another at the house and provide copies to trusted friends if you wish. Besides written copies of your advance directives, be sure to speak with your loved ones and answer their questions so they understand your wishes.[R56]

Accomplish unfinished tasks: There are a few other things you can do to help yourself bring a sense of meaning and completion to your life. Is there a trip you were dreaming of achieving, but cancer stopped you from pursuing such a dream? Fund-raising can help. Is there a book you want to read? Do you wish to spend time with specific individuals, resolve conflict, or to say goodbye to some people? These wishes, dreams, and circumstances may include solving disagreements, a farewell to select individuals, and telling members of the family how much you love them. If you can't talk, consider writing, calling, or sending a message through a relative.

Assess your life: Consider taking time to reflect on and commemorate your life, including the things you've accomplished with individuals you've loved, and the occasions that have formed you. Talk to your friends and family about the special times you have invested together. You'll commend the life you shared and create brand-new memories for them to value.

Stories can correspond to gifts to the people you'll leave behind. As you examine your life, you might wish to compose or record your memories or ask somebody to write for you as you talk. Sharing your aspirations and dreams for loved ones may help ease your heartache and concern about leaving them behind. It also helps them feel connected to you at select times in their lives. For young children, you may allow them to have videos and albums that remind them of your love and connection.

Go back to religion: Religion is an essential part of life for some people where the support of faith and clergy members is a significant source of comfort at the end of life. Others may discover spiritual solace in nature or people. As you ready yourself, seek involvement that brings a sense of convenience, peace, meaning, and completion. Patients and their families must feel comfortable asking their healthcare team to help find spiritual support.

FOR CAREGIVERS AND FAMILY MEMBERS

Often, those closest to the patient, like caregivers and family members, receive most of the patient's anger. It's natural since the patient feels safest with these people knowing that they won't be disappointed with him or her for being angry. Calming down and talking about it benefits the patient by reducing anger. Caregivers and family members must realize that the patient's animosity is natural, and they must try to ease this anger to the best of their ability. Telling the patient he or she isn't a burden, and they did their best in the past and talking about good times may lower the effects of regret and guilt.

Being together enables relatives to support each other. Even though you have gathered, please don't assume it suggests you'll be there at the end. The individual doesn't pass away until those who were present have left. It's like they can't let go when loved ones are still there. The author of *Final Journeys: A Practical Guide for Bringing Care and Comfort at the End of Life*, who has witnessed over two thousand deaths said, "Dying people have the uncanny ability to choose the moment of death, and it's not uncommon for them to spare those they love the most or feel protective of by waiting until those people leave the room."

Ignoring the fact that facing the reality of one's death raises the difficulty many individuals have when it's time to communicate with dying individuals. Research has shown that not being able to handle the intensity of the situation or not having the time to become involved are the main reasons for some individuals to abstain from communicating with a dying individual. For some people, grieving is a factor, and for loved ones, it's the belief whether they could somehow prevent their loved one's death giving rise to personal guilt that causes them to avoid communication with their dying loved one. Despite the circumstances forbidding such contact, family members should try to discount their feelings and talk to the dying person.

Saying goodbye is tricky even when spoken to a small child on the way to school. Saying goodbye to a loved one dying of cancer is overwhelming. It will leave you with scars, but going through it propels you forward and assist you in grieving. Although the process starts with devastation and fear, it will end with acceptance. Part of that process will include bidding farewell. If you preserve a keen focus on the individual you love, you'll get through it more easily. Focus on saying what you think they need to hear about attaining peace. The goodbye aims to leave you both in harmony.

When bidding farewell, it's essential to state things you won't look back on later with regret. Plan and rehearse what you'll say and investigate your heart to explore the ideal words.

As a caregiver or a family member, putting off a meaningful conversation with your dying loved one is a source of regret. Don't wait to say what's on your mind, disclose your affection and appreciation, and be thankful for your loved one's presence in your life, tell them positive things you know they want to hear. Don't wait to say goodbye; it may be too late. Don't insist that the person will get well; it's comforting to neither of you, the truth is you must face reality, show up and be with the dying person, you're his world just by being there, hold hands if you can. Throw in a joke here and there, laughter is great for everyone, and it will give the dying person some peace within and help ignore the situation even if only for a few minutes, it's also all right to cry.

Honesty isn't always the very best policy. If you have a family issue and on your dad's deathbed, he asks you to promise to solve it after he's gone, it's vital to say you'll do everything you can to see through to resolve the matter. Let him opt for hope by stating things that promote peace. While it's challenging to make this happen, if you have challenging siblings and you have dysfunctional relations with them, try to keep that out of sight throughout this farewell.

CONCLUSION

I love to read cancer survivor's stories, especially when the outcomes are excellent. I am also a member of many cancer organizations and cancer social media groups where patients post short stories about their experiences with diagnosis and treatment, and how they choose to cope. Regretfully, a high number of survivors appear to have given up on the disease. One survivor posted, "Never tell me what, when, and how to eat, I'll kill you." These types of situations give me a sense of unhappiness, and it's very disappointing even to imagine that a patient would think in this manner, but I don't blame them. Many who show signs of desperation think that cancer will kill them.

We are *all* unique human beings, and we think about life differently, especially when the issue at hand is sickness. We cope with situations from our perspective on life, how we're raised, our strengths and weaknesses and a multitude of other factors. But despite how you manipulate a problem, you can never change reality. You can only work hard to improve specific outcomes.

Yes, cancer is dreadful, and it can definitely kill you, but what you must understand is that it isn't a death sentence anymore. We have accomplished and progressed so much with cancer research in the past two decades, where some survivors now would never have dreamed of being alive today compared to the past. Despite the dreadful nature of cancer, it can be treated and contained in a large number of situations. But to control this beast you must have the tools necessary to do so.

Research tells us that quitting smoking, controlling our weight, and protecting ourselves from infections such as the HPV through vaccination can significantly reduce our exposure to cancer; public health would improve overnight, and cancer incidence would fall dramatically and improve immediately.

By changing behaviors, you can eliminate or reduce many of these factors and minimize the risk of cancer. Although this knowledge seems to favor a preventive side, the information is vital to improving your health while living with, through, or beyond cancer. The three main risk factors are critical in controlling your tumor by shrinking its size and helping prevent metastasis and recurrence throughout your survivorship journey.

You didn't choose to have cancer. But now you have it, and you must make choices to reach the results you want. Your decisions can only be more effective when accompanied by hope and optimism. Don't abandon your past life just because you have cancer. Learn from the past and use the knowledge you gained for your benefit. Can you envision some of those impossible situations in your past? Do you remember what you had to do to solve them? Enhance those solutions and apply them to your current situation.

Learn about your disease, execute a well-prepared case-specific survivorship plan, and follow up on it faithfully under the continued supervision of your oncologist. This will make you the best person to manage your condition as a chronic illness. As a survivor, you have encountered many events during your cancer journey. They are landmarks that reshaped your life and made you unique and proud; you can tackle the most difficult situations.

I hope that *Cancer Survivorship: How to Navigate the Turbulent Journey* has helped you to make the right choices about your survivorship, including treatment and finding your new normal. Making the right decisions will lead you to live with less pain and give you the peace of mind to search for your health needs to sustain a healthy life. I hope you found that luminous landing strip after a long and troublesome storm.

My wish is for every cancer patient to start understanding that our bodies react to cancer differently. Sharing a cancer type, even the stage, with someone else doesn't mean that the outcomes will be the same. You may have horrible cancer, but you may also recover. Cancer can be treated. Advances in medicine and technology are progressing at astronomical speeds, and fresh, new scientific minds are arriving enthusiastically to spread the good news. This book gave you the tools to succeed. Now go out there and use them. Never underestimate what you can accomplish when you believe in yourself.

Never give up.

ACKNOWLEDGMENTS

I want to thank the almighty God for enabling me to research and write on a complex subject and for giving me the strength not to quit. Thank you for giving me the patience and the opportunity to help others.

This book has developed out of a series of interactions with cancer patients spanning over two decades. Writing this book would not have been possible without witnessing the courage, confidence, and strength my patients showed me during their journeys. They proved that despite the destructive nature of cancer, it's still manageable when backed by knowledge and persistence. They showed me that one could attain the possible from the impossible. Franklin D. Roosevelt once said, "When you come to the end of the rope, tie a knot and hang on." These patients tied a knot at the end of the rope and held on to it with strength instead of giving up and slipping. To all my past and present patients: thank you for being great teachers.

I can't express enough thanks to the professionals at the American Cancer Society and the National Cancer Institute, including all their oncologists, nurses, administrative personnel, and volunteers for answering a million questions without a breath of hesitation. And thank you for answering questions I did not ask.

I want to express my deep and sincere gratitude to all my crew at Cancerhall, especially, Ms. Kelly Thompson, who dedicated her precious time to making hundreds of calls on behalf of this book. Kelly, you're an inspiration.

To all those oncologists, counselors, nutritionists, and naturopathic doctors who received my questions with open arms, allow me to say thank you for your patience and kindness in helping and addressing my concerns.

Finally, I am grateful to my family and friends for their love, prayers, and caring and for pushing me to complete this project. A special thanks to my best friend, Shadi Al-Musa, for giving me his undivided attention every time I conversed with him about this book.

Shadi, I want you to know that I listened to every suggestion you tried to deliver, although I may have seemed to ignore you. Completing this book was possible because of your continued support and encouragement. Your friendship means everything to me. I also want you to know that I will need your exceptional help when I write my next book, which, God willing, will be soon.

BIBLIOGRAPHY

"3 Tips for Transitioning Out of Cancer Treatment." Cancer.Net, July 15, 2019. https://www.cancer.net/blog/2017-09/3-tips-transitioning-out-cancer-treatment.

"5 Steps to Help You Make Cancer Treatment Decisions." Mayo Clinic. Mayo Foundation for Medical Education and Research, April 25, 2019. https://www.mayoclinic.org/diseases-conditions/cancer/in-depth/cancer-treatment/art-20047350.

"6 Tips for Recognizing Milestones in a Life with Cancer." Cancer.Net, May 15, 2019. https://www.cancer.net/blog/2016-04/6-tips-recognizing-milestones-life-with-cancer.

"A Change of Work Priorities." Cancer & Work. Accessed December, 20, 2018. https://www.cancerandwork.ca/healthcare-providers/assisting-patients-in-changing-work-looking-for-work/a-change-of-work-priorities/.

"A Doctor Asks: What Does a Cancer Coach Do?" Cancer Harbors, May 17, 2016. https://cancerharbors.com/cancer-coach/.

Abdoler, Emily, Holly Taylor, and David Wendler. "The Ethics of Phase 0 Oncology Trials." Clinical Cancer Research. American Association for Cancer Research, June 15, 2008. https://clincancerres.aacrjournals.org/content/14/12/3692.

"About Clinical Trials." Cancer.Net, September 30, 2018. https://www.cancer.net/research-and-advocacy/clinical-trials/about-clinical-trials.

Abrahm, Janet L. *Physicians Guide to Pain and Symptom Management in Cancer Patients*. Johns Hopkins University Press, 2015.

Adami, Hans-Olov, David J. Hunter, Pagona Lagiou, Lorelei A. Mucci, and Brian MacMahon. *Textbook of Cancer Epidemiology*. New York: Oxford University Press, 2018.

Adler, Elizabeth M. *Living with Lymphoma: A Patients Guide*. Johns Hopkins University Press, 2016.

Alschuler, Lise, Karolyn A. Gazella, and Lise Alschuler. *The Definitive Guide to Cancer: An Integrative Approach to Prevention, Treatment, and Healing*. Berkeley, CA: Ten Speed, 2010.

Alschuler, Lise, Karolyn A. Gazella, and Lise Alschuler. *The*

Definitive Guide to Cancer: An Integrative Approach to Prevention, Treatment, and Healing. Ten Speed, 2010.

Amin, Mahul B., Stephen B. Edge, and Frederick L. Greene. *AJCC Cancer Staging Manual.* Cham: Springer, 2017.

Anderson, Greg, and Greg Anderson. *Cancer: 50 Essential Things to Do.* New York: Plume, 2013.

Anekwe, Tobenna D., and Ilya Rahkovsky. "Self-Management: A Comprehensive Approach to Management of Chronic Conditions." *American Journal of Public Health* 108, no. S6 (2018). https://doi.org/10.2105/ajph.2014.302041r.

Bannasch, Peter. *Cancer Diagnosis: Early Detection.* Berlin: Springer, 1992.

Barnard, Neal. *Cancer Survivors Guide: Foods That Help You Fight Back!* Book Publishing Company, 2017.

Becton, Randy. *Everyday Strength: A Cancer Patients Guide to Spiritual Survival.* Baker Books, 2006.

Beer, Tomasz M., and Larry Axmaker. *Cancer Clinical Trials: Your Commonsense Guide to Experimental Cancer Therapies and Clinical Trials.* Amistad, 2012.

Benish, Shannon R. *How to Help Someone with Cancer: 70 Ways to Help Cancer Patients and Their Families during Cancer Treatment.* Place of publication not identified: Rebel Redd Books, 2017.

Bevell, Brett. *Reiki for Spiritual Healing.* Random House USA, 2009.

Béliveau Richard. *Foods to Fight Cancer: Essential Foods to Help Prevent Cancer.* DK, 2017.

Bien, Thomas, and Beverly Bien. *Mindful Recovery: A Spiritual Path to Healing from Addiction.* J. Wiley & Sons, 2002.

Bollinger, Ty M. *Truth About Cancer: What You Need to Know About Cancers History, Treatment, And Prevention.* Place of Publication Not Identified: Hay House Inc, 2018.

Bollinger, Ty M. *Cancer: Step Outside the Box.* McKinney, TX: Infinity 510^2 Partners, 2014.

Boxer, Harriet, and Susan Snyder. "Five Communication Strategies to Promote Self-Management of Chronic Illness." Family Practice Management, October 1, 2009. https://www.aafp.org/fpm/2009/0900/p12.html.

Boyd, D. Barry., and Marian Betancourt. *The Cancer Recovery Plan: Maximize Your Cancer Treatment with This Proven Nutrition, Exercise, and*

Stress-Reduction Program. Avery, 2005.

Breitbart, William, and Shannon R. Poppito. *Individual Meaning-Centered Psychotherapy for Patients with Advanced Cancer: A Treatment Manual*. New York, NY: Oxford Univ. Press, 2014.

Buddeberg, Claus. "Psychosocial Support and Problems in Cancer Patients." *Supportive Care in Cancer*2, no. 4 (1994): 209–. https://doi.org/10.1007/bf00365722.

Burgess, Rob. *Stem Cells: A Short Course*. Wiley Blackwell, 2016.

Bush, Nancy Jo, and Linda M. Gorman. *Psychosocial Nursing Care along the Cancer Continuum*. Pittsburgh, PA: Oncology Nursing Society, 2018.

"Cancer." World Health Organization. World Health Organization. Accessed November 29, 2018. https://www.who.int/news-room/fact-sheets/detail/cancer.

Cancer Australia. "The Cancer Experience: The Person Diagnosed with Cancer." EdCaN. Cancer Australia, November 25, 2014. http://edcan.org.au/edcan-learning-resources/supporting-resources/cancer-journey/cancer-experience.

"Cancer Clinical Trials." Cancer Research Institute. Accessed January 19, 2019. https://www.cancerresearch.org/patients/clinical-trials.

Cancer Connect. "Managing Side Effects of Cancer Treatment." news.cancerconnect.com. Cancer Connect, April 22, 2019. https://news.cancerconnect.com/treatment-care/managing-side effects-of-cancer-treatment-zeg-ivtUFkaNusI3tXOBeg/.

"Cancer Pain (Cancer Symptoms) Information: MyVMC." HealthEngine Blog, March 21, 2019. https://healthengine.com.au/info/cancer-pain-2.

"Cancer Pain: Relief Is Possible." Mayo Clinic. Mayo Foundation for Medical Education and Research, November 3, 2018. https://www.mayoclinic.org/diseases-conditions/cancer/in-depth/cancer-pain/art-20045118.

"Cancer Side Effect Management and Depression." Cancer Treatment Centers of America, February 17, 2019. https://www.cancercenter.com/integrative-care/depression.

"Cancer Survivorship." American Nurse Today, April 7, 2017. https://www.americannursetoday.com/cancer-survivorship/.

"Cancer Treatment: Know Your Options." EverydayHealth.com, February 9, 2010.

https://www.everydayhealth.com/cancer/understanding/treatment-methods.aspx.

"Cancer Treatments." CancerQuest. Accessed January 07, 2019. https://www.cancerquest.org/patients/treatments.

"Cancer: What Scientists Know Vs. What the Public Believes." Office for Science and Society, May 30, 2018. https://www.mcgill.ca/oss/article/health-general-science/cancer-what-scientists-know-versus-what-public-believes.

"Care Through the Final Days." Cancer.Net, July 12, 2019. https://www.cancer.net/navigating-cancer-care/advanced-cancer/care-through-final-days.

Caring for Patients Across the Cancer Care Continuum. Place of Publication Not Identified: Springer, 2019.

Carmona, Richard H., and Mark Liponis. *Integrative Preventive Medicine*. Oxford University Press, 2018.

Carr, Allen. *The Easy Way to Stop Smoking*. New York: Sterling, 2004.

Chabner, Bruce, and Dan L. Longo. *Cancer Chemotherapy, Immunotherapy, and Biotherapy: Principles and Practice*. Wolters Kluwer, 2019.

Chambers, David A., Cynthia A. Vinson, and Wynne E. Norton. *Advancing the Science of Implementation across the Cancer Continuum*. New York, NY: Oxford University Press, 2019.

"Changes in Physical Appearance and Body Image." Cancer & Work. Accessed September 30, 2018. https://www.cancerandwork.ca/healthcare-providers/cancers-impact-on-work/effects-physical/.

"Changing Priorities." LIVESTRONG, November 17, 2016. https://www.livestrong.org/we-can-help/feelings-emotions/changing-priorities.

"Choices for Care with Advanced Cancer." National Cancer Institute. Accessed January 13, 2019. https://www.cancer.gov/about-cancer/advanced-cancer/care-choices.

Chopra, Deepak. *The Seven Spiritual Laws of Yoga: A Practical Guide to Healing Body, Mind*. John Wiley & Sons, 2005.

"Clinical Trials." Millennium Physicians. Accessed September 20, 2019. https://millenniumphysicians.com/clinical-trials/.

"Clinical Trials for Cancer." Cancer Support Community, So that No One Faces Cancer Alone. Accessed January 19, 2019.

https://www.cancersupportcommunity.org/clinical-trials-cancer.

Cooper, Geoffrey M. "The Development and Causes of Cancer." The Cell: A Molecular Approach. 2nd edition. US National Library of Medicine, January 1, 1970. https://www.ncbi.nlm.nih.gov/books/NBK9963/.

"Counting the Ways Life Will Be Better after Cancer." dummies. Accessed January 22, 2019. https://www.dummies.com/health/diseases/cancer/counting-the-ways-life-will-be-better-after-cancer/.

Cuomo, Margaret I. *World without Cancer: The Making of a New Cure and the Real Promise of Prevention.* New York: Rodale, 2013.

Dale, Teri. *I Refused Chemo: 7 Steps to Taking Back Your Power & Healing Your Cancer.* New York: Morgan James Publishing, 2018.

Daudt, H. M. L., C. Van Mossel, D. L. Dennis, L. Leitz, H. C. Watson, and J. J. Tanliao. "Survivorship Care Plans: A Work in Progress." *Current Oncology* 21, no. 3 (2014): 466. https://doi.org/10.3747/co.21.1781.

Davis, Carol M., and Gina Maria Musolino. *Patient Practitioner Interaction: An Experiential Manual for Developing the Art of Health Care.* Thorofare, NJ: SLACK Incorporated, 2016.

Demicheli, R., M. W. Retsky, W. J. M. Hrushesky, M. Baum, and I. D. Gukas. "The Effects of Surgery on Tumor Growth: A Century of Investigations." *Annals of Oncology* 19, no. 11 (2008): 1821–28. https://doi.org/10.1093/annonc/mdn386.

Desaulniers Véronique. *Heal Breast Cancer Naturally: 7 Essential Steps to Beating Breast Cancer.* TCK Publishing, 2014.

Downing, Nancy. "What a Cancer-Free Declaration by Your Doctor Really Means." The Truth About Cancer, May 13, 2016. https://thetruthaboutcancer.com/what-cancer-free-means/.

Duff, Nancy J. *Making Faithful Decisions at the End of Life.* Westminster John Knox Press, 2018.

Dulaney, Caleb, Audrey S Wallace, Ashlyn S Everett, Laura Dover, Andrew Mcdonald, and Lauren Kropp. "Defining Health Across the Cancer Continuum." *Cureus*, 2017. https://doi.org/10.7759/cureus.1029.

East, Cara. "Strategies for Cancer Survivorship: Practical Advice from a Doctor and Patient." *Baylor University Medical Center Proceedings* 13, no. 1 (2000): 14–18. https://doi.org/10.1080/08998280.2000.11927637.

Eeles, Rosalind A., Christine D. Berg, and Jeffrey S. Tobias. *Cancer Prevention and Screening: Concepts, Principles and Controversies*. Hoboken, NJ: John Wiley & Sons, Inc., 2019.

Eib, Lynn. *Finding the Light in Cancers Shadow*. Tyndale House Publishers, 2006.

Eldridge, Lynne. "How to Advocate for Yourself as a Cancer Patient." Verywell Health. Verywell Health, June 24, 2019. https://www.verywellhealth.com/how-to-be-your-own-advocate-as-a-cancer-patient-2248881.

"Embracing Mind, Body and Spirit in the Treatment of Cancer." Cancer Knowledge Network, April 17, 2013. https://cancerkn.com/embracing-mind-body-and-spirit-in-the-treatment-of-cancer/.

"Emotional & Physical Effects." MD Anderson Cancer Center. Accessed January 02, 2019. https://www.mdanderson.org/patients-family/diagnosis-treatment/emotional-physical-effects.html.

"Emotions After Cancer Treatment." LIVESTRONG, October 3, 2016. https://www.livestrong.org/we-can-help/finishing-treatment/emotions-after-cancer-treatment.

"Emotions and Coping as You Near the End of Life." American Cancer Society. Accessed December 23, 2018. https://www.cancer.org/treatment/end-of-life-care/nearing-the-end-of-life/emotions.html.

"End-of-Life Care." National Cancer Institute. Accessed March 20, 2019. https://www.cancer.gov/about-cancer/advanced-cancer/care-choices/care-fact-sheet.

"Ethical Considerations for Phase 1 Clinical Trials." ASCO Connection, April 6, 2015. https://connection.asco.org/magazine/current-controversies-oncology/ethical-considerations-phase-1-clinical-trials.

"For Patients & Families." Dana. Accessed April 02, 2019. https://www.dana-farber.org/for-patients-and-families/for-survivors/caring-for-yourself-after-cancer/medical-care-after-treatment/.

"For Patients & Families." Dana. Accessed January 12, 2019. https://www.dana-farber.org/for-patients-and-families/for-survivors/caring-for-yourself-after-cancer/your-body-after-treatment/.

"For Patients & Families." Dana. Accessed January 17, 2019.

https://www.dana-farber.org/for-patients-and-families/for-survivors/caring-for-yourself-after-cancer/developing-a-wellness-plan/.

Foster, C, and D Fenlon. "Recovery and Self-Management Support Following Primary Cancer Treatment." *British Journal of Cancer*105, no. S1 (2011). https://doi.org/10.1038/bjc.2011.419.

Frank, Steven A. "Multistage Progression." Dynamics of Cancer: Incidence, Inheritance, and Evolution. US National Library of Medicine, January 1, 1970. https://www.ncbi.nlm.nih.gov/books/NBK1562/.

Friedman, Lawrence M., Curt D. Furberg, David L. DeMets, David M. Reboussin, and Christopher B. Granger. *Fundamentals of Clinical Trials*. Springer International Publishing, 2015.

Frähm, David J. *A Cancer Battle Plan Sourcebook: A Step-by-Step Health Program to Give Your Body a Fighting Chance*. J. P. Tarcher/Putnam, 2000.

Ganz, Patricia A. "The 'Three Ps' of Cancer Survivorship Care." BMC medicine. BioMed Central, February 10, 2011. https://www.ncbi.nlm.nih.gov/pmc/articles/PMC3060853/.

Gardner, Kirsten E. *Early Detection: Women, Cancer, & Awareness Campaigns in the Twentieth-Century United States*. Chapel Hill: University of North Carolina Press, 2006.

Geense, Wytske W, Irene M Van De Glind, Tommy Ls Visscher, and Theo Van Achterberg. "Barriers, Facilitators and Attitudes Influencing Health Promotion Activities in General Practice: An Explorative Pilot Study." *BMC Family Practice*14, no. 1 (September 2013). https://doi.org/10.1186/1471-2296-14-20.

Geist, Laura, and Susan Sorensen. *Praying through Cancer: Set Your Heart Free from Fear, a 90-Day Devotional for Women*. Thomas Nelson, 2006.

Gerson, Charlotte. *Gerson Therapy: The Proven Nutritional Program to Fight Cancer and Other Illnesses*. Kensington Pub Corp, 2001.

Gilbert, Scott M., David C. Miller, Brent K. Hollenbeck, James E. Montie, and John T. Wei. "Cancer Survivorship: Challenges and Changing Paradigms." *Journal of Urology*179, no. 2 (2008): 431–38. https://doi.org/10.1016/j.juro.2007.09.029.

Gknation. "Long-Term and Late Effects for Cancer Survivors." Long-Term and Late Effects for Cancer Survivors | Leukemia and Lymphoma Society, February 26, 2015.

https://www.lls.org/managing-your-cancer/long-term-and-late-effects-for-cancer-survivors.

"Goals of Cancer Treatment." QualityCancerTreatment.com. Accessed April 20, 2019. https://www.qualitycancertreatment.com/know-the-goals-of-cancer-treatment.html.

Grimm, Peter, John Blasko, and John Sylvester. *The Prostate Cancer Treatment Book*. New York: McGraw-Hill, 2004.

Gruman, Jessie C. *Cancer Survivorship: What I Wish Id Known Earlier*. Center for Advancing Health, 2013.

Guntupalli, Saketh R., and Maryann Karinch. *Sex and Cancer: Intimacy, Romance, and Love after Diagnosis and Treatment*. Lanham, MD: Rowman & Littlefield, 2017.

Gutkind, Lee, and Francine Prose. *At the End of Life: True Stories about How We Die*. Creative Nonfiction, 2012.

Gwynn, Cat. *10-Mile Radius: Reframing Life on the Path through Cancer*. Rare Bird Books, 2017.

Haddad, Laura Holmes. *This Is Cancer: Everything You Need to Know, from the Waiting Room to the Bedroom*. Seal Press, 2016.

Hall, Eric J., and Amato J. Giaccia. *Radiobiology for the Radiologist*. Wolters Kluwer, 2019.

Harpham, Wendy S. *When a Parent Has Cancer: A Guide to Caring for Your Children*. HarperCollins e-books, 2011.

Harpham, Wendy S., and Emma C. Mathes. *Healing Hope: through and beyond Cancer*. Currant house, 2018.

Horan, Anthony H. *How to Avoid the Over-Diagnosis and Over-Treatment of Prostate Cancer*. Broomfield, CO: On the Write Path Publishing, 2012.

"Hospice Care." Cancer.Net, January 23, 2019. https://www.cancer.net/navigating-cancer-care/advanced-cancer/hospice-care.

"How Cancer Starts, Grows and Spreads - Canadian Cancer Society." www.cancer.ca. Accessed November 20, 2018. http://www.cancer.ca/en/cancer-information/cancer-101/what-is-cancer/how-cancer-starts-grows-and-spreads/?region=on.

"How Has Cancer Changed Your Life?" Fifth Season Financial, March 31, 2016. https://www.fifthseasonfinancial.com/blog/how-has-cancer-changed-your-life/.

Hudson, Melissa M. "A Model for Care across the Cancer

Continuum." Wiley Online Library. John Wiley & Sons, Ltd, October 28, 2005. https://onlinelibrary.wiley.com/doi/full/10.1002/cncr.21250.

Hudson, S. V., S. M. Miller, J. Hemler, J. M. Ferrante, J. Lyle, K. C. Oeffinger, and R. S. Dipaola. "Adult Cancer Survivors Discuss Follow-up in Primary Care: Not What I Want, But Maybe What I Need." *The Annals of Family Medicine*10, no. 5 (January 2012): 418–27. https://doi.org/10.1370/afm.1379.

IHadCancer.com. "I've Reached My 5-Year Cancerversary. Now What?" Cancer Support Community for Peer to Peer Help. Accessed September 20, 2019. https://www.ihadcancer.com/h3-blog/12-28-2015/i've-reached-my-5-year-cancerversary-now-what.

"Infertility: Radiation Therapy Side Effects." Cancer Council NSW. Accessed February 17, 2019. https://www.cancercouncil.com.au/cancer-information/cancer-treatment/radiation-therapy/side effects/infertility/.

Irwin, Melinda L. *ACSMs Guide to Exercise and Cancer Survivorship*. Human Kinetics, 2012.

Johnson Memorial Health. "The Important Role of Volunteers in Today's Hospitals." The Important Role of Volunteers in Today's Hospitals. Accessed December 13, 2018. https://blog.johnsonmemorial.org/the-important-role-of-volunteers-in-todays-hospitals.

Katz, Anne. *Surviving after Cancer: Living the New Normal*. Rowman & Littlefield, 2012.

Katz, Barbara. *Connecting Care for Patients: Interdisciplinary Care Transitions and Collaboration*. Burlington, MA: Jones & Bartlett Learning, 2020.

"Key Components of Survivorship Care." ASCO, August 30, 2019. https://www.asco.org/practice-guidelines/cancer-care-initiatives/prevention-survivorship/survivorship/survivorship.

Kralik, Debbie, Tina Koch, Kay Price, and Natalie Howard. "Chronic Illness Self-Management: Taking Action to Create Order." *Journal of Clinical Nursing*13, no. 2 (2004): 259–67. https://doi.org/10.1046/j.1365-2702.2003.00826.x.

"Late Effects of Childhood Cancer Treatment." American Cancer Society. Accessed January 07, 2019. https://www.cancer.org/treatment/children-and-cancer/when-your-child-has-cancer/late-effects-of-cancer-treatment.html.

"Learn to Control the Nausea and Vomiting That Come with Chemo." WebMD. WebMD. Accessed February 15, 2019. https://www.webmd.com/cancer/holistic-treatment-17/cut-chemo-side effects.

Leong, Stanley P. L. *Cancer Clinical Trials: Proactive Strategies.* Springer Science Business Media, LLC, 2007.

"Life After Cancer." American Cancer Society. Accessed September 20, 2019. https://www.cancer.org/treatment/survivorship-during-and-after-treatment/be-healthy-after-treatment/life-after-cancer.html.

"Life after Treatment." Life after cancer treatment | Cancer Council Victoria. Accessed March 03, 2019. https://www.cancervic.org.au/living-with-cancer/life-after-treatment/living-well-after-cancer.

"Life Isn't the Same: How Cancer Changes You." Roswell Park Comprehensive Cancer Center. Accessed March 22, 2019. https://www.roswellpark.org/cancertalk/201612/life-isnt-same-how-cancer-changes-you.

"Long-Term Side Effects of Cancer Treatment." Cancer.Net, May 17, 2019. https://www.cancer.net/survivorship/long-term-side effects-cancer-treatment.

Longtin, Yves, Hugo Sax, Lucian L. Leape, Susan E. Sheridan, Liam Donaldson, and Didier Pittet. "Patient Participation: Current Knowledge and Applicability to Patient Safety." *Mayo Clinic Proceedings* 85, no. 1 (2010): 53–62. https://doi.org/10.4065/mcp.2009.0248.

Majumder, Sadhan. *Stem Cells and Cancer.* Springer, 2009.

"Making a Treatment Decision That Is Right for You." Cancer Support Community, So that No One Faces Cancer Alone. Accessed September 20, 2019. https://www.cancersupportcommunity.org/OpentoOptions.

"Making Decisions About Cancer Treatment." Cancer.Net, July 25, 2019. https://www.cancer.net/navigating-cancer-care/how-cancer-treated/making-decisions-about-cancer-treatment.

"Making Decisions with Your Doctor." National Institute on Aging. US Department of Health and Human Services. Accessed January 09, 2019. https://www.nia.nih.gov/health/making-decisions-your-doctor.

"Managing Cancer as a Chronic Illness." American Cancer

Society. Accessed January 17, 2019. https://www.cancer.org/treatment/survivorship-during-and-after-treatment/when-cancer-doesnt-go-away.html.

"Managing Cancer-Related Side Effects." American Cancer Society. Accessed December 11, 2018. https://www.cancer.org/treatment/treatments-and-side effects/physical-side effects.html.

"Managing Physical Side Effects." Cancer.Net. Accessed February 01, 2019. https://www.cancer.net/coping-with-cancer/physical-emotional-and-social-effects-cancer/managing-physical-side effects/dry-mouth-or-xerostomi.

"Managing the Lingering Side Effects of Cancer Treatment." Mayo Clinic. Mayo Foundation for Medical Education and Research, February 19, 2019. https://www.mayoclinic.org/diseases-conditions/cancer/in-depth/cancer-survivor/art-20045524.

Marston, Dianna Mitchell. *Living with Cancer as "a New Normal": A Journey with Cancer through the Eyes of a Caregiver.* iUniverse, Inc., 2007.

Mccorkle, Ruth, Elizabeth Ercolano, Mark Lazenby, Dena Schulman-Green, Lynne S. Schilling, Kate Lorig, and Edward H. Wagner. "Self-Management: Enabling and Empowering Patients Living with Cancer as a Chronic Illness." *CA: A Cancer Journal for Clinicians*61, no. 1 (2011): 50–62. https://doi.org/10.3322/caac.20093.

Mccorkle, Ruth, Elizabeth Ercolano, Mark Lazenby, Dena Schulman-Green, Lynne S. Schilling, Kate Lorig, and Edward H. Wagner. "Self-Management: Enabling and Empowering Patients Living with Cancer as a Chronic Illness." *CA: A Cancer Journal for Clinicians*61, no. 1 (2011): 50–62. https://doi.org/10.3322/caac.20093.

Mcdermott, Patrick Orton Colin. *Physics and Technology of Radiation Therapy.* Medical Physics Publishing, 2018.

McIntosh, J. Richard. *Understanding Cancer: An Introduction to the Biology, Medicine, and Societal Implications of This Disease.* Boca Raton: CRC Press, Taylor & Francis Group, 2019.

McKay, Judith, and Tamera Schacher. *The Chemotherapy Survival Guide: Everything You Need to Know to Get through Treatment.* New Harbinger Publications, 2009.

McKinney, Neil. *Naturopathic Oncology: An Encyclopedic Guide for*

Patients & Physicians. Liaison Press, 2016.

McLean, Bonnie. *Integrative Medicine: The Return of the Soul to Healthcare*. Balboa Press, a division of Hay House, 2015.

"Memory Loss and Concentration after Cancer Treatment." Irish Cancer Society, January 16, 2017. https://www.cancer.ie/support/coping-with-cancer/life-after-cancer-treatment/memory-loss-and-concentration.

"Men with Cancer Are Less Likely to Accept Palliative Care." Futurity, July 9, 2018. https://www.futurity.org/palliative-care-men-1804872-2/.

Michaelson, Jessica. "Self-Nurture: A Prerequisite to Self-Care." DrJessicaMichaelson. DrJessicaMichaelson, December 21, 2015. http://www.drjessicamichaelson.com/blog/self-nurture.

Mil José van, Christine Archer-Mackenzie, and Henk Brandsen. *Healthy Eating during Chemotherapy: For the First Time, a Chef and a Medical Specialist Have Teamed Up to Inspire You with over 100 Delicious Recipes*. Kyle Books, 2019.

"Models of Long-Term Follow-Up Care." ASCO, November 30, 2016. https://www.asco.org/practice-guidelines/cancer-care-initiatives/prevention-survivorship/survivorship/survivorship-3.

Morewitz, Stephen J. *Chronic Diseases and Health Care*. New York: Springer Science Business Media, Inc., 2006.

Murshed, Hasan. *Fundamentals of Radiation Oncology: Physical, Biological, and Clinical Aspects*. Amsterdam: Academic Press, 2019.

Nagourney, Robert A. *Outliving Cancer: The Better, Smarter, Faster Way to Treat Cancer*. Basic Health, 2013.

Nathan, David G. *The Cancer Treatment Revolution: How Smart Drugs and Other New Therapies Are Renewing Our Hope and Changing the Face of Medicine*. Hoboken, NJ: John Wiley & Sons, 2007.

National Academies of Sciences, Engineering and Medicine, Health and Medicine Division, Board on Health Care Services, National Cancer Policy Forum, Sharyl J. Nass, Margie Patlak, and Erin Balogh. *Incorporating Weight Management and Physical Activity Throughout the Cancer Care Continuum Proceedings of a Workshop*. Washington, D.C: National Academies Press, 2018.

"National Comprehensive Cancer Network." Finding Comfort in Spirituality. Accessed December 20, 2018. https://www.nccn.org/patients/resources/life_with_cancer/spirituality.aspx.

"National Comprehensive Cancer Network." Mood Changes Associated with Cancer Treatment. Accessed February 13, 2019. https://www.nccn.org/patients/resources/life_with_cancer/managing_symptoms/mood_changes.aspx.

"National Comprehensive Cancer Network." Managing Cancer as a Chronic Condition, n.d. https://www.nccn.org/patients/resources/life_after_cancer/managing.aspx.

"NCI Dictionary of Cancer Terms." National Cancer Institute. Accessed December 11, 2018. https://www.cancer.gov/publications/dictionaries/cancer-terms/def/survivorship.

"Neglecting Mental Health in Cancer Treatment." Psychology Today. Sussex Publishers. Accessed April 05, 2019. https://www.psychologytoday.com/us/blog/nurturing-self-compassion/201702/neglecting-mental-health-in-cancer-treatment-0.

Neustatter, Patrick. *Managing Your Doctor: The Smart Patients Guide to Getting Effective Affordable Healthcare*. North Charleston, SC: CreateSpace Independent Publishing Platform, 2015.

"New Options in Androgen Therapy." Cure Today. Accessed April 05, 2019. https://www.curetoday.com/publications/cure/2010/winter2010/New-Options-in-Androgen-Therapy.

Noé Jody E., and Peter D'Adamo. *Textbook of Naturopathic Integrative Oncology*. CCNM Press, 2012.

"Oncolink." Oncolink. Accessed April 06, 2019. https://oncolife.oncolink.org/.

Ornish, Dean, and Anne Ornish. *Undo It!: How Simple Lifestyle Changes Can Reverse Most Chronic Diseases*. Ballantine Books, 2019.

Osborne, Helen. *Overcoming Communication Barriers in Patient Education*. Gaithersburg, MD: Aspen Publishers, 2001.

Parrott, Roxanne. *Talking about Health: Why Communication Matters*. Chichester, U.K: Wiley-Blackwell, 2009.

Phiri, Violet, Nikos Chamitzidis, Enrico Bagayawa, Susan Arnott, Diane Pitts, Janet Newham, Cruzan Sheldon, et al. "Cancer—Why Some Get It and Some Don't." The Truth About Cancer, May 31, 2017. https://thetruthaboutcancer.com/cancer-get-dont/.

Pierce, Tanya Harter. *Outsmart Your Cancer: Alternative Non-Toxic Treatments That Work*. Thoughtworks Pub., 2009.

"Planning the Transition to End-of-Life Care in Advanced Cancer (PDQ®)–Health Professional Version." National Cancer Institute, n.d. https://www.cancer.gov/about-cancer/advanced-cancer/planning/end-of-life-hp-pdq.

Pothier, Kristin Ciriello. *Personalizing Precision Medicine: A Global Voyage from Vision to Reality*. John Wiley & Sons, Inc., 2017.

Precision Cancer Medicine: Challenges and Opportunities. Springer, 2019.

Press, The Associated. "When to Give up: Treatment or Comfort for Late-Stage Cancer?" National Post, June 6, 2016. https://nationalpost.com/health/when-to-give-up-treatment-or-comfort-for-late-stage-cancer.

Prochaska, James O., and Janice M. Prochaska. *Changing to Thrive: Using the Stages of Change to Overcome the Top Threats to Your Health and Happiness*. Hazelden Publishing, 2016.

Purtilo, Ruth B., Amy Marie. Haddad, and Regina F. Doherty. *Health Professional and Patient Interaction*. St. Louis, MO: Elsevier, 2014.

"Questions to Ask about Cancer Treatment Clinical Trials." National Cancer Institute. Accessed May 20, 2019. https://www.cancer.gov/about-cancer/treatment/clinical-trials/questions.

Research. "Hair Loss (Alopecia) From Radiation Treatment." OncoLink. Accessed May 21, 2019. https://www.oncolink.org/support/side effects/skin-hair-nail-side effects/hair-loss-alopecia-from-radiation-treatment.

"Research Areas: Screening and Early Detection." National Cancer Institute. Accessed November 13, 2018. https://www.cancer.gov/research/areas/screening.

"Resources for Survivors." Memorial Sloan Kettering Cancer Center. Accessed January 14, 2019. https://www.mskcc.org/experience/living-beyond-cancer/resources-survivors.

"Returning to a Normal Life after Cancer." Cancer Council NSW, July 10, 2017. https://www.cancercouncil.com.au/15289/b1000/living-well-after-cancer-45/living-well-after-cancer-back-to-normal/.

Roby, Mark. *Lifelines to Cancer Survival: A New Approach to Personalized Care*. Integrative Medicine Publishing, 2015.

Rosenbaum, Ernest H. *Everyone's Guide to Cancer Survivorship: A Road Map for Better Health*. Andrews McMeel Pub., 2007.

Ryan, Michele. *Cancer: What I Wish I Had Known When I Was First Diagnosed: Tips and Advice from a Survivor*. North Charleston, SC: CreateSpace, 2014.

Scotting, Paul, and Kelly Birch. *Cancer*. United States: Oneworld Publications, 2017.

"Seasons of Survivorship." Cure Today. Accessed January 30, 2019. https://www.curetoday.com/publications/cure/2009/fall-supplement2009/seasons-of-survivorship.

Servan-Schreiber, David. *Anticancer: A New Way of Life*. NY, NY: Penguin Books, 2017.

Shapiro, Rick. *Hope Never Dies: How 20 Late-Stage and Terminal Cancer Patients Beat the Odds: Including Exclusive Interviews with 5 Renowned Cancer Specialists: How They Are Saving Lives Now*. Innovative Healing Press, LLC, 2017.

"Side effects of Radiation Therapy for Cancer Treatment." WebMD. WebMD. Accessed February 1, 2019. https://www.webmd.com/cancer/what-to-expect-from-radiation-therapy#1.

"Signs of Dying from Cancer." Crossroads Hospice Expect more from us. We do. Accessed March 11, 2019. https://www.crossroadshospice.com/hospice-caregiver-support/end-of-life-signs/cancer/.

"Spirituality in Cancer Care (PDQ®)–Patient Version." National Cancer Institute. Accessed April 12, 2019. https://www.cancer.gov/about-cancer/coping/day-to-day/faith-and-spirituality/spirituality-pdq.

Stengler, Mark. *Outside the Box Cancer Therapies: Alternative Therapies That Treat and Prevent Cancer*. Hay House, Inc., 2018.

"Steps to Successful Self-Management of Your Emotional State." The Coaching Academy, n.d. https://www.the-coaching-academy.com/blog/steps-to-successful-self-management-of-your-emotional-state-534.asp.

"Symptoms of Cancer." National Cancer Institute. Accessed May 15, 2019. https://www.cancer.gov/about-cancer/diagnosis-staging/symptoms.

Synopsis of Key Gynecologic Oncology Trials. CRC Press, 2019.

Tako, Barbara. *Cancer Survivorship Coping Tools - We'll Get You through This: Tools for Cancers Emotional Pain from a Melanoma and Breast Cancer Survivor.* Ayni Books, 2015.

Templeton, James. *I Used to Have Cancer.* Square One Pub, 2019.

"The Importance of Follow-Up Care." Cancer.Net, June 28, 2019. https://www.cancer.net/survivorship/follow-care-after-cancer-treatment/importance-follow-care.

"The Importance of Social Support When Diagnosed with Cancer." healthpsychologynow, n.d. http://www.healthpsychologynow.com/social-support-cancer.html.

"The Placebo Effect: What Is It?" WebMD. WebMD. Accessed November 10, 2018. https://www.webmd.com/pain-management/what-is-the-placebo-effect#1.

Thompson, R. Paul, and Ross E. G. Upshur. *Philosophy of Medicine: An Introduction.* Routledge, 2018.

"Types of Cancer." Cancer Research UK, December 5, 2017. https://www.cancerresearchuk.org/what-is-cancer/how-cancer-starts/types-of-cancer#carcinomas.

"Understanding Maintenance Therapy." Cancer.Net, May 29, 2019. https://www.cancer.net/navigating-cancer-care/how-cancer-treated/understanding-maintenance-therapy.

UPMC. "Scar Care After Surgery: Minimizing Scarring." UPMC HealthBeat, August 29, 2019. https://share.upmc.com/2017/11/scar-care-after-surgery/.

UpToDate. Accessed June 19, 2019. https://www.uptodate.com/contents/complementary-and-alternative-medicine-treatments-cam-for-cancer-beyond-the-basics.

Vahdat, Shaghayegh, Leila Hamzehgardeshi, Somayeh Hessam, and Zeinab Hamzehgardeshi. "Patient Involvement in Health Care Decision Making: A Review." *Iranian Red Crescent Medical Journal* 16, no. 1 (May 2014). https://doi.org/10.5812/ircmj.12454.

Varona, Verne. *Natures Cancer-Fighting Foods: Prevent and Reverse the Most Common Forms of Cancer Using the Proven Power of Whole Food and Self-Healing Strategies.* Viking, 2014.

Vickers, Elaine. *A Beginners Guide to Targeted Cancer Treatments.* Hoboken: Wiley, 2018.

"Volunteering and Its Surprising Benefits." HelpGuide.org, July 15, 2019. https://www.helpguide.org/articles/healthy-living/volunteering-and-its-surprising-benefits.htm.

Wagener, C., Carol Stocking, and Müller Oliver. *Cancer Signaling:*

from Molecular Biology to Targeted Therapy. Weinheim: Wiley-VCH Verlag GmbH & Co. KGaA, 2017.

Walter and Miller's Textbook of Radiotherapy: Radiation Physics, Therapy And. S.L.: Elsevier Health Sciences, 2019.

Walter and Miller's Textbook of Radiotherapy: Radiation Physics, Therapy And. S.L.: Elsevier Health Sciences, 2019.

Weiner, Reina S. *Trust Your Doctor... but Not That Much: Be Your Own Best Healthcare Advocate.* Place of publication not identified: Why Wait, LLC., 2019.

Weiner, Reina S. *Trust Your Doctor... but Not That Much: Be Your Own Best Healthcare Advocate.* Place of publication not identified: Why Wait, LLC., 2019.

Weiss, Marisa C., and Ellen Weiss. *Living Well Beyond Breast Cancer: A Survivors Guide for When Treatment Ends and the Rest of Your Life Begins.* New York, USA: Crown, 2010.

"What Are Cancer Clinical Trials?" National Cancer Institute. Accessed January 19, 2019. https://www.cancer.gov/about-cancer/treatment/clinical-trials/what-are-trials.

"What Are the Phases of Clinical Trials?" American Cancer Society. Accessed February 11, 2019. https://www.cancer.org/treatment/treatments-and-side effects/clinical-trials/what-you-need-to-know/phases-of-clinical-trials.html.

"What Can I Do About Cancer Pain? What Are the Treatments?" WebMD. WebMD. Accessed November 18, 2018. https://www.webmd.com/cancer/cancer-pain-what-helps#1.

"What Comes After Finishing Treatment: An Expert Q&A." Cancer.Net, July 25, 2019. https://www.cancer.net/survivorship/life-after-cancer/what-comes-after-finishing-treatment-expert-qa.

"What Is a Cancer Research Advocate?" Cancer.Net, December 13, 2016. https://www.cancer.net/blog/2016-12/what-cancer-research-advocate.

"What Is Cancer Recurrence?" American Cancer Society. Accessed March 20, 2019. https://www.cancer.org/treatment/survivorship-during-and-after-treatment/understanding-recurrence/what-is-cancer-recurrence.html.

"What to Know about Surgery for Cancer." Mayo Clinic. Mayo Foundation for Medical Education and Research, July 9, 2019.

https://www.mayoclinic.org/diseases-conditions/cancer/in-depth/cancer-surgery/art-20044171.

"What?! Cancer Survivorship Has Stages?!?" Sherry Strong, September 21, 2018. https://www.sherrystrong.org/cancer-survivorship-stages/.

"When Surgery Is the Best Cancer Treatment." EverydayHealth.com, February 9, 2010. https://www.everydayhealth.com/cancer/when-surgery-is-the-best-treatment.aspx.

Wiestler, Otmar D., Bernhard Haendler, and Dominik Mumberg. *Cancer Stem Cells*. Springer-Verlag Berlin Heidelberg, 2007.

Wolfelt, Alan, and Kirby J. Duvall. *Healing Your Grieving Heart after a Cancer Diagnosis: 100 Practical Ideas for Coping, Surviving, and Thriving*. Companion Press, 2014.

Yokota, and Jun. "Tumor Progression and Metastasis." OUP Academic. Oxford University Press, March 1, 2000. https://academic.oup.com/carcin/article/21/3/497/2365673.

Zucchermaglio, Cristina, and Francesca Alby. "Social Interactions and Cultural Repertoires as Resources for Coping with Breast Cancer - Cristina Zucchermaglio, Francesca Alby, 2017." SAGE Journals. Accessed September 20, 2019.

Zwahlen, Diana. *Families Facing Cancer*. Place of publication not identified: Sudwestdeutscher Verlag F, 2011.

RESOURCES

The following collection of resources is a list of well-known and trusted cancer organizations dedicated to serving cancer patients everywhere. They are comprised of professionals and well-trained volunteers to answer all your questions and help through your cancer journey. They are capable of addressing your concerns concerning any topic related to cancer. They can also provide you with a list of cancer organizations, hospitals, cancer clinics, counselors, coaches, and oncology physical therapists in your local area. If you're newly diagnosed with cancer, ask for brochures and information on your cancer situation. You can always ask for more information as you navigate through your journey.

The following set of resources is divided into two broad categories: general cancer resources and topic-specific cancer resources.

GENERAL CANCER RESOURCES

1. **National Coalition for Cancer Survivorship**
   8455 Colesville Road, Suite 930
   Silver Spring, MD 20910
   877-NCCS-YES
   info@canceradvocacy.org
   Website: Caceradvocacy.org

2. **The National Cancer Institute**
   BG 9609 MSC 9760
   9609 Medical Center Drive
   Bethesda, MD 20892-9760
   Website: Cancer.gov

3. **American Cancer Society**
   250 Williams Street NW
   Atlanta, GA 30303
   Website: Cancer.org
   Phone Number: 1-800-227-2345

4. **American Institute for Cancer Research**
   PO Box 97167
   Washington, DC 20090-7167
   Administrative Office
   1560 Wilson Boulevard Suite 1000
   Arlington, VA 22209
   Telephone: 1-800-843-8114
   aicrweb@aicr.org
   Website: aicr.org

5. **CancerCare**
   275 Seventh Avenue
   New York, NY1000
   Telephone number:1800-813-HOPE (4673)
   info@cancercare.org
   Website: Cancercare.org

6. **Journey Forward**
   Website: Journeyforward.org

7. **CancerHall Survivor Network**
   Cancerhall.com

8. **Live Strong**
   2201 E. Sixth Street
   Austin, TX 78702
   Telephone number: 1-855-220-7777
   Website: livestrong.org

9. **National Cancer Survivors Day**
   P.O. Box 682285
   Franklin, TN 37068-2285
   Telephone number: 1-615-794-3006
   Website: ncsd.org

10. **American Society of Clinical Oncology (ASCO)**
    2318 Mill Road, Suite 800, Alexandria, VA 22314
    Email: contactus@cancer.net
    1-571-483-1780 or 1-888-651-3038
    Website: Cancer.net

11. **St. Jude Children's Research Hospital (Childhood Cancer)**
    262 Danny Thomas Place
    Memphis, TN 38105
    1 -866-278-5833
    Website: stjude.org

RESOURCES ABOUT SPECIFIC CANCER TOPICS

The following list of resources is topic-specific. You can use them to gather detailed information about your cancer including how to self-manage your cancer at any stage of the disease. Some of the listed resources contain addresses and phone numbers, and all of them contain a specific reference to a web page address to particular topics included in this book.

12. **Navigating the Cancer Continuum**
    http://s3.amazonaws.com/pfizerpro.com/assets/patientnavigation.com/Patient_Navigation_in_Cancer_Care_2.0_%C2%ADWebsite_12.04.18.pdf

13. **Defining Health across the Continuum**
    US National Library of Medicine
    National Institute of Health
    9000 Rockville Pike
    Bethesda, Maryland 20892
    301-496-4000
    TTY 301-402-9612
    https://www.ncbi.nlm.nih.gov/pmc/articles/PMC5354402/

14. **Cancer Care on the Continuum**
    https://www.medicaldosimetry.org/default/assets/File/roswell2016/Mack_Noelle.pdf

15. **Cancer Basics**
    MedlinePlus
    US National Library of Medicine
    8600 Rockville Pike
    Bethesda, MD 20894
    https://medlineplus.gov/cancer.html

16. **Types of Cancer**
    Cancer Support Community
    734 15th Street NW | Suite 300
    Washington, DC 20005
    Cancer Helpline: 888-793-9455
    Phone: 202-659-9709
    https://www.cancersupportcommunity.org/learn-about-cancer-types

17. **Cancer Causes**
    NCBI

https://www.ncbi.nlm.nih.gov/books/NBK54025/#targetText=The%20three%20leading%20types%20of,cancer%20incidence%20in%20developing%20countries.

18. **Cancer Treatment**
    MD Anderson Cancer Center
    https://www.mdanderson.org/patients-family/diagnosis-treatment/treatment-options.html

    Mayo Clinic
    201 W. Center St.
    Rochester, MN 55902
    1-507-266-7890

    Chemocare
    1-844-268-3901
    chemocare@ccf.org

    Cancer Center
    1-844-334-8116

19. **Cancer Symptoms**
    Emedicinehealth
    https://www.emedicinehealth.com/cancer_symptoms/article_em.htm#what_should_i_know_about_cancer

20. **Cancer Prognosis**
    Canadian Cancer Society
    55 St Clair Avenue West, Suite 500
    Toronto, Ontario M4V 2Y7
    1-888-939-3333
    https://www.cancer.ca/en/cancer-information/cancer-101/what-is-cancer/prognosis-and-survival/?region=on

21. **Cancer Remission**
    Healthline
    660 Third Street
    San Francisco, CA 94107
    1-415-281-3100

    New York Office
    275 Seventh Ave., 24th Floor
    New York, NY 10001
    1-917-720-4400
    https://www.healthline.com/health/cancer/cancer-remission#diagnosing-remission

US National Library of Medicine
National Institute of Health
8600 Rockville Pike
Bethesda, MD 20894
1-800-422-6237
https://www.ncbi.nlm.nih.gov/pmc/articles/PMC4754119/

22. **Why Do Most People Never Get Cancer?**
Medical Xpress
https://medicalxpress.com/news/2009-01-majority-people-cancer.html

23. **Cancer Clinical Trials**
Cancer Center
1-977-505-6130
https://www.cancercenter.com/clinical-trials

National Cancer Institute
8600 Rockville Pike
Bethesda, MD 20894
1-800-422-6237
https://www.cancer.gov/about-cancer/treatment/clinical-trials

National Institute on Aging
Building 31, Room 5C27
31 Center Drive, MSC 2292
Bethesda, MD 20892
1-800-222-2225
1-800-438-4380
https://www.nia.nih.gov/health/clinical-trials-benefits-risks-and-safety

Safety in clinical trials
US National Library of Medicine
ClinicalTrials.gov

24. **Alternative and Complementary Medicine**
Johns Hopkins Medicine
1-410-955-5000
https://www.hopkinsmedicine.org/health/wellness-and-prevention/types-of-complementary-and-alternative-medicine

National Center for Complementary and Integrative Health
9000 Rockville Pike
Bethesda, Maryland 20892
1-888-644-6226
https://nccih.nih.gov/health/integrative-health

MedicineNet

https://www.medicinenet.com/alternative_medicine/article.htm#tocb

25. **Placebo Effect**
Harvard Medical School
Harvard Health Publishing
4 Blackfan Circle, 4th Floor
Boston, MA 02115 USA
https://www.health.harvard.edu/mental-health/the-power-of-the-placebo-effect

Cancer Research UK- Safety in Alternative and Complementary Medicine
0808-800-4040
https://www.cancerresearchuk.org/about-cancer/cancer-in-general/treatment/complementary-alternative-therapies/about/safety

26. **Specialized Cancer Care—Palliative Care**
National Institute on Aging
Building 31, Room 5C27
31 Center Drive, MSC 2292
Bethesda, MD 20892
1-800-222-2225
https://www.nia.nih.gov/health/what-are-palliative-care-and-hospice-care

Get Palliative Care
https://getpalliativecare.org/what-is-palliative-chemotherapy/
https://getpalliativecare.org/whatis/disease-types/breast-cancer-palliative-care/
https://getpalliativecare.org/whatis/disease-types/cancer-palliative-care/

National Cancer Institute
1-800-422-6237
https://www.cancer.gov/about-cancer/advanced-cancer/care-choices/palliative-care-fact-sheet#targetText=Palliative%20care%20is%20care%20given,whole%2C%20not%20just%20their%20disease.

American Society of Clinical Oncology (ASCO)
Cancer.net
https://www.cancer.net/coping-with-cancer/physical-emotional-and-social-effects-cancer/what-palliative-care

The American Cancer Society
250 Williams Street NW
Atlanta, GA 30303
Website: Cancer.org
1-800-227-2345

https://www.cancer.org/treatment/treatments-and-side effects/palliative-care.html

27. **Specialized Cancer Care—Hospice Care**
    MedlinePlus
    https://medlineplus.gov/hospicecare.html

    MedicineNet
    US National Library of Medicine
    8600 Rockville Pike
    Bethesda, MD 20894
    https://www.medicinenet.com/script/main/art.asp?articlekey=24267

28. **Cancer Diagnosis**
    Stanford Health Care
    1-800-756-9000
    https://stanfordhealthcare.org/medical-conditions/cancer/cancer/cancer-diagnosis.html

    American Society of Clinical Oncology (ASCO)
    Cancer.net
    https://www.cancer.net/navigating-cancer-care/diagnosing-cancer/tests-and-procedures

29. **Dealing with Diagnosis Shock**
    Medical News Today
    130 Queens Road, First Floor
    Brighton, East Sussex, BN1 3WB. United Kingdom
    011 44-845-468-0075
    https://www.medicalnewstoday.com/articles/319749.php

    Canadian Cancer Society
    1-888-939-3333
    https://www.cancer.ca/en/cancer-information/cancer-journey/recently-diagnosed/?region=on

30. **Understanding the Cancer Pathology Report**
    Texas Oncology
    Texasoncology.com
    https://www.texasoncology.com/cancer-treatment/surgery/understanding-your-pathology-report

    Susan G. Komen
    5005 LBJ Freeway
    Suite 526
    Dallas, TX 75244
    1-877-465-6636

https://ww5.komen.org/BreastCancer/ContentsofaPathologyReport.html

American Cancer Society
250 Williams Street NW
Atlanta, GA 30303
Website: Cancer.org
1-800-227-2345
https://www.cancer.org/treatment/understanding-your-diagnosis/tests/understanding-your-pathology-report.html

31. **Navigating Cancer Treatments**
American Society of Clinical Oncology (ASCO)
Cancer.net
https://www.cancer.net/navigating-cancer-care/how-cancer-treated/making-decisions-about-cancer-treatment

STAT
1 Exchange Place, Suite 201
Boston, MA 02109-2132
https://www.statnews.com/2017/12/14/cancer-treatment-decision-making/

US National Library of Medicine
National Institute of Health
8600 Rockville Pike
Bethesda, MD 20894
https://www.ncbi.nlm.nih.gov/pmc/articles/PMC2913835/

Journal of Oncology Practice
American Society of Clinical Oncology (ASCO)
2318 Mill Road, Suite 800
Alexandria, VA 22314
https://ascopubs.org/doi/full/10.1200/jop.2014.001434

National Cancer Institute
1-800-422-6237
https://www.cancer.gov/about-cancer/treatment/questions

32. **Stopping Cancer Treatment**
Verywell Health
1500 Broadway
New York, NY 10036
212-204-4000
https://www.verywellhealth.com/when-should-you-stop-cancer-treatment-2249017

33. **After Cancer Treatment**
    Cancer Support Community
    734 15th Street NW | Suite 300
    Washington, DC 20005
    Cancer Helpline: 888-793-9355
    202-659-9709
    https://www.cancersupportcommunity.org/resources

34. **Financial Resources**
    American Society of Clinical Oncology (ASCO)
    Cancer.net
    https://www.cancer.net/navigating-cancer-care/financial-considerations/financial-resources

    National Cancer Institute
    1-800-422-6237
    https://www.cancer.gov/resources-for/patients

35. **Psychological Resources**
    Dana-Farber Cancer Institute
    450 Brookline Avenue
    Boston, MA 02215
    https://www.dana-farber.org/adult-psychosocial-oncology/

    Clinical Advances in Hematology & Oncology
    CAHO@dmdconnects.com
    https://www.hematologyandoncology.net/archives/december-2016/the-management-of-psychological-issues-in-oncology/

    American Psychological Association
    750 First St. NE
    Washington, DC 20002-4242
    1-800-374-2721
    1-202-336-5500
    https://www.apa.org/monitor/2014/11/emotions-cancer

36. **Spiritual Resources**
    National Comprehensive Cancer Network
    3025 Chemical Road, Suite 100, Plymouth Meeting, PA 19462 •
    215.690.0300
    https://www.nccn.org/patients/resources/life_with_cancer/spirituality.aspx

    US National Library of Medicine
    National Institute of Health
    8600 Rockville Pike

Bethesda, MD 20894
https://www.ncbi.nlm.nih.gov/pmc/articles/PMC4332130/

37. **Social Resources**
Cancer Financial Assistance Coalition
https://www.cancerfac.org/

OHSU Knight Cancer Institute
1-503-494-8311
https://www.ohsu.edu/knight-cancer-institute/cancer-patient-and-family-resources

Disability Benefits Help
1-833-251-8797
https://www.disability-benefits-help.org/disabling-conditions/cancer-and-social-security-disability#targetText=Cancer%20and%20Social%20Security%20Disability,qualifications%20may%20be%20more%20straightforward.

38. **Adapting to Health after Treatment**
Harvard Health Publishing
4 Blackfan Circle, 4th Floor
Boston, MA 02115 USA
https://www.health.harvard.edu/cancer/adapting-to-life-after-cancer

Cancer Council
153 Dowling Street, Woolloomooloo NSW 2011
Cancercouncil.com.au
https://www.cancercouncil.com.au/15289/b1000/living-well-after-cancer-45/living-well-after-cancer-back-to-normal/

National Cancer Institute
1-800-422-6237
https://www.cancer.gov/publications/patient-education/facing-forward

Mayo Clinic
1-480-301-8000
https://www.mayoclinic.org/diseases-conditions/cancer/in-depth/cancer-survivor/art-20044015
City of Hope
1500 East Duarte Road
Duarte, CA 91010
1-626-256-4673
https://www.cityofhope.org/nutrition-after-cancer-treatment/

National Comprehensive Cancer Network
3025 Chemical Road, Suite 100

Plymouth Meeting, PA 19462
1-215-690-0300
https://www.nccn.org/patients/resources/life_with_cancer/exercise.aspx

39. **Knowing More About Cancer Survivorship**
    The National Academies of Science Engineering Medicine
    500 Fifth St., NW
    Washington, DC 20001
    https://www.nap.edu/read/11468/chapter/4

    US National Library of Medicine
    National Institute of Health
    8600 Rockville Pike
    Bethesda, MD 20894
    https://www.ncbi.nlm.nih.gov/pmc/articles/PMC6516397/

40. **Cancer Remission**
    Healthline
    660 Third Street
    San Francisco, CA 94107
    1-415-281-3100
    https://www.healthline.com/health/cancer/cancer-remission

    Dignity Health
    Dignityhealth.org
    https://www.dignityhealth.org/articles/treatment-terminology-remission-meaning-vs-cancer-free

    Verywell Health
    1500 Broadway
    New York, NY 10036
    212-204-4000
    https://www.verywellhealth.com/what-does-cancer-remission-mean-2249186

    CancerConnect
    Cancerconnect.com
    https://news.cancerconnect.com/treatment-care/frequently-asked-questions-about-the-role-of-maintenance-therapy-in-cancer-XKb2IavFRECXHxnpt2T8hw/

    Dana-Farber Cancer Institute
    450 Brookline Avenue
    Boston, MA 02215
    1-617-632-3000
    https://blog.dana-farber.org/insight/2018/12/mean-remission-cancer/

41. **Cancer as a Chronic Illness**
    National Comprehensive Cancer Network
    3025 Chemical Road, Suite 100
    Plymouth Meeting, PA 19462 • 215.690.0300
    1-215-690-0300
    https://www.nccn.org/patients/resources/life_after_cancer/managing.aspx

42. **Cancer Coping**
    National Cancer Institute
    1-800-422-6237
    https://www.cancer.gov/about-cancer/coping

43. **Survivorship Planning**
    American Cancer Society
    250 Williams Street NW
    Atlanta, GA 30303
    Website: Cancer.org
    Phone Number: 1-800-227-2345

    Cancer.org
    https://www.cancer.org/treatment/survivorship-during-and-after-treatment/survivorship-care-plans.html

    Memorial Sloan Kettering Cancer Center
    1275 York Avenue
    New York, NY 10065
    1-212-639-2000
    https://www.mskcc.org/hcp-education-training/survivorship/survivorship-care-plan

44. **Making Adjustments After Cancer**
    US National Library of Medicine
    8600 Rockville Pike
    Bethesda, MD 20894
    https://www.ncbi.nlm.nih.gov/pmc/articles/PMC4503227/

45. **Nurturing the Body, Mind, and Soul**
    Psych Central
    55 Pleasant St., Suite 207
    Newburyport, MA
    01950https://blogs.psychcentral.com/weightless/2018/03/how-to-deeply-nurture-yourself/

46. **Cancer Coaching**
    Cancer Harbors

https://cancerharbors.com/cancer-coach/

47. **Cancer Volunteering and Advocacy**
American Society of Clinical Oncology (ASCO)
1-888-651-3038
1-571-483-1780
Cancer.net
https://www.cancer.net/blog/2017-12/how-cope-with-cancer-through-volunteering

Cancer Support Community
734 15th Street NW | Suite 300
Washington, DC 20005
Cancer Helpline: 1-888-793-9355
1-202-659-9709
https://www.cancersupportcommunity.org/volunteer

American Cancer Society
250 Williams Street NW
Atlanta, GA 30303
Website: Cancer.org
1-800-227-2345
https://www.cancer.org/about-us/what-we-do/advocacy.html

48. **Late Effects of Cancer**
Livestrong
2201 E. Sixth Street
Austin, TX 78702
1-855-220-7777
https://www.livestrong.org/we-can-help/healthy-living-after-treatment/late-effects-of-cancer-treatment

Mayo Clinic
507-538-3270
https://www.mayoclinic.org/diseases-conditions/cancer/in-depth/cancer-survivor/art-20045524

Canadian Cancer Society
1-888-939-3333
https://www.cancer.ca/en/cancer-information/cancer-journey/life-after-cancer/late-and-long-term-effects-of-treatment/?region=on

49. **Cancer Recurrence**
Cancer Therapy Advisor
275 7th Avenue, 10th Floor
New York, NY 10001

https://www.cancertherapyadvisor.com/home/tools/fact-sheets/cancer-recurrence-statistics/

Susan G. Komen
5005 LBJ Freeway
Suite 526
Dallas, TX 75244
1-877-465-6636
https://ww5.komen.org/BreastCancer/SurvivalandRiskofHavingCancerReturnAfterTreatment.htm

50. **Second Cancers**
National Comprehensive Cancer Network
3025 Chemical Road, Suite 100
Plymouth Meeting, PA 19462
1-215-690-0300
https://www.nccn.org/patients/resources/life_after_cancer/understanding.aspx

Journey Forward
Journeyforward.org
https://www.journeyforward.org/document/second-cancers-adults

51. **Life's Meaning**
Psychology Today
Psychologytoday.com
https://www.psychologytoday.com/us/blog/hide-and-seek/201803/what-is-the-meaning-life

MM.net
Markmanson.net
https://markmanson.net/the-meaning-of-life

52. **Finding a New Normal**
Cancer Council
153 Dowling Street
Woolloomooloo NSW 2011
https://www.cancercouncil.com.au/15289/b1000/living-well-after-cancer-45/living-well-after-cancer-back-to-normal/
Aurora Health Care
750 W. Virginia St
P.O. Box 341880
Milwaukee, Wisconsin 53204
https://www.aurorahealthcare.org/patients-visitors/blog/after-beating-cancer-whats-next-the-new-normal

MD Anderson Cancer Center

1-855-384-6254
https://www.mdanderson.org/publications/cancerwise/adjusting-to-the-new-normal.h00-158753112.html

53. Moving Forward
Cure
Curetoday.com
https://www.curetoday.com/community/bonnie-annis/2016/06/life-after-cancer-learning-to-move-forward

54. End-of-Life Period
Crossroads Hospice & Palliative Care
1-855-327-4677
https://www.crossroadshospice.com/hospice-caregiver-support/end-of-life-signs/

Pallimed
Pallimed.org
https://www.pallimed.org/2017/12/the-emotions-of-dying.html

Cancer Research UK
0808-800-4040
https://www.cancerresearchuk.org/about-cancer/coping/dying-withcancer/last-few-weeks-and-days/final-days

Cancer Council
615 St Kilda Road,
Melbourne, Victoria, 3004, Australia
61 3 9514 6100
https://www.cancervic.org.au/get-support/facing-end-of-life/caring-for-someone-nearing-the-end-of-life

Healthline
660 Third Street
San Francisco, CA 94107
1-415-281-3100
New York Office
275 Seventh Ave., 24th Floor
New York, NY 10001
https://www.healthline.com/health/signs-of-death

American Cancer Society
250 Williams Street NW
Atlanta, GA 30303
Website: Cancer.org
1-800-227-2345

https://www.cancer.org/treatment/end-of-life-care/nearing-the-end-of-life/death.html

55. **Bereavement Services**
    Hospice Patients Alliance
    Hospicepatients.org
    https://hospicepatients.org/hospic11.html

    High Peaks Hospice
    1-518-891-0606
    http://highpeakshospice.org/bereavement-care/

56. **Advance Directives**
    MedlinePlus
    US National Library of Medicine
    8600 Rockville Pike
    Bethesda, MD 20894
    https://medlineplus.gov/advancedirectives.html

    MedicineNet
    Medicinenet.com

GREAT CANCER HOSPITALS

There are hundreds of excellent cancer hospitals and clinics across the nation. Below is a list of the top hospitals. If you need a more extensive list, consult with the National Cancer Institute and the American Cancer Society. Don't forget to get a full professional background about your oncologist(s).

MD Anderson Cancer Canter
1-866-971-6253
Mdanderson.org

Memorial Sloan Kettering
212-639-2000
Mskcc.org

The Mayo Clinic
507-284-2511
Mayoclinic.org

Dana-Farber Cancer Institute
617-632-3000
Dana-farber.org

Cleveland Clinic Cancer Center
800-223-2273
My.clevelandclinic.org

The Sidney Kimmel Comprehensive Cancer Center
Oncology Department
410-955-8980
Hopkinsmedicine.org

Seattle Cancer Care Alliance
855-557-0555
Website seatlecca.org

Moffitt Cancer Center
1-888-663-3488
Website: moffitt.org

UCSF Helen Diller Family Comprehensive Cancer Center
888-689-8273
Cancer.ucsf.edu

Abramson Cancer Center
800-789-7366
Pennmedicine.org

ABOUT THE AUTHOR

Hussam Haj Hasan is a health physicist, a cancer researcher, and the director of Cancerhall Survivor Network, CSN. He taught modern and radiation physics to science and medical students in various universities in the United States and abroad. He has performed his doctoral research on the risks and benefits associated with radiation to protect public health and the environment. A few years after completing his doctoral work, he wanted to further his academic ambitions to pursue a career in cancer prevention and education. He used his prior training in physics to serve as a basis to advocate for an interdisciplinary approach to more effective cancer research, a critical approach to helping doctors to implement resources from other scientific disciplines to strengthen their pursuit of finding a cancer cure or at least reduce the mortality rate.

He founded Cancerhall Survivor Network in 1993 with the primary aim of encouraging cancer patients to make health decisions through collaboration with their doctors. This cooperation is necessary to pursue optimal health and is only possible through educating the patient. Cancerhall started offering online cancer-related courses for nonpatients and case-specific education for patients in 2012.

His work involves managing a national database composed of experienced cancer professionals, including oncologists, counselors, coaches, nutritionists, oncology physical therapists, certified integrative medicine practitioners, and cancer support centers. Please check our website, www.cancerhall.com. Upon joining, patients are matched with professionals from the database in their geographic locations where the choice of experts depends on the patient's cancer situation requirements. Before the selection process begins, Cancerhall's staff perform case-analysis, navigate treatment options, and offer the necessary education to the patient. The case study results are further embedded in an assessment report and submitted to the designated cancer professionals to resume the survivorship planning and support. Cancerhall supervises the entire process and offers the support needed for the professionals and the patients to ensure that there are no obstacles to effective communication and to make certain that the patients receive the best care.

INDEX

A

abdominal area, 172, 177
    pain in the, 30
abdominal cavities, 19
abnormal cells, 29, 157
acceptance, 91, 145, 199-203
active dying, 196
acupuncture, 48, 56, 151
acute pain, 150
acute phase, 8, 76
    of survivorship, 74
acute, 8, 90, 127
adaptation, 140
addiction, fear of, 151
adenocarcinoma, 19, 28
adjustments, 118, 137
    health, 120, 142
    lifestyle, 79, 92
    making the, 122-127
    physical, 142, 147-151
    psychological, 143-147
    to the new environment, 108
adjuvant therapy, 26
admittance eligibility, 42
adoptive cell transfer, 24
adrenal glands, 176
advance directives, 61, 200-201
advanced stage, 30, 104
advances in cancer treatment
    and research, 4, 27, 33, 69
advice, 5, 58, 76-77, 88, 110
    doctor's, 68, 105, 151
    financial, 93
Advil, 150
advocacy, 159-162
    cancer, 161
    group, 44
aggressive, 18, 32, 61

cancer, 37, 61, 74, 152
    testing, 31
    therapies, 104
alcohol, 34, 68, 89
    follow-up plan and, 140
    mouthwashes that contain, 178
    prevention and, 6
    stop or reduce drinking, 126
    stress and, 89
allogeneic transplants, 27
alternative medicine, 46-47, 51-53, 57
    categories of, 52
    considering, 54
    costs of, 55-56
    effectiveness of, 46
    favoring, 54
    safety issues in, 53-54
    who pays for, 55
American Academy of Hospice
    and Palliative Medicine, 67
American Board of Medical
    Specialties, 110
American Cancer Society, 7, 51, 96, 111-126, 133
American College of Surgeons, 110-111
American Medical Association, 110
American Psychological Association, 113
American Society of Clinical
    Oncology, 61
amputation, 150
analyze, 152, 185
anemia, 27, 148, 171, 173
anesthesia, 21, 175
anger, 194
antibodies, 24
anticancer, 53
    drugs, 4
    therapy, 48
antidepressants, 151
antioxidants, 53
anxiety, 119
    diagnosis and, 89-90
    distress and, 113
    hypnotherapy and, 48

massage therapy and, 48-49
meditation and, 49
music therapy and, 49
relaxations technique and, 50
risky behaviors and, 89
social support and, 116-117
spirituality and, 113-116
treatment for, 62, 90, 112
yoga and, 49
appetite, 159
    changes in, 30, 173, 196
    loss of, 91
artery, 24, 174
arthritis, 175, 180
aspirations, 202
aspirin, 150
assisted living, 200
assisted-care facility, 63
asymptomatic, 78, 168-169
attitude, 189
    positive, 127-128, 156
audiologist, 174
autologous transplants, 26
Ayurveda, 52

B

balance, 8, 80, 145
    cell, 17
    diet, 124-125
barriers, 7, 152
belief in God, 116
benign, 18, 97, 169
bereavement care and services, 14, 65
bidding farewell, 203
biofeedback, 93
biological therapy, 24, 102
biological, 52, 54, 157
biomedical signals, 158
biopsy, 21, 94-95
bladder, 24, 30
blame, 88, 92
bleeding, 27, 30, 102, 180
blockage, 30
blood cells, 19, 24, 27
blood clots, 25-27, 31

blood in the stool, 180
blood loss, 23
blood pressure, 25-26, 88, 115, 125
blood sugar level, 88
blood tests, 133
blood transfusion, 23
blood vessels, 19, 22, 30, 126
bloodstream, 18, 31, 172
board certified, 110
bodily disfigurement, 144
body image, 121
body parts, 76, 121
bone damage, 27
bone marrow, 19
    transplants, 26, 148
bone problems, *see* osteoporosis
bones, 19-27, 148, 175
brachytherapy, 23, 102
brain changes, 174
brain tumor, 7
brain, 17, 19, 28, 30, 119
    activities, 173
    chemical changes in the, 145
    radiation directed at the, 177
    tumors, 7
breast cancer, 26, 48
    and yoga, 49
breastbone, 172
breathing, 197
    and relaxation, 93
    and tai chi, 49
    changes in, 196
    congested, 196
    deep, 49, 93, 145
    devices, 201
    strategies, 157-158
    trouble, 25, 178

C

bruising, 180
caffeine, 125, 145, 178
calcium level, 31
calories, 125, 173
CAM, 47-58, 142
cancer advocacy, 161-162
    see also advocacy

cancer centers, 111
cancer coaching, 159-160
    see also coaching
cancer treatments, 9, 33, 101, 119
    advances in, 33
    chemotherapy, 24
    conventional, 49, 53
    hormone therapy, 26
    immunotherapy, 24-25
    precision medicine, 27
    pros and cons of, 101
    radiation therapy, 23
    specific, 67
    stem cell transplant, 26-27
    surgery, 21-23
    targeted therapy, 25-26
cancer:
    basics, 12, 77
    causes of, 20–23
    clinical trials, 12, 36-45
    definition of, 17-19
    development of, 17-18
    diagnosis, 85-97
    diet and, *see* nutrition
    early-screening, 7
    emotional impact of, 4, 15, 33, 86-90, 143-147
    environmental factors and, 21, 34
    financial impact of, 6, 7
    fundamentals, 12, 15-35
    future of your, 31-34
    growth of, 17-27
    hair loss and, 121, 174-176
    histology of your, 140
    incurable, 138
    lifeline, 5
    organizations, 94
    origination, 12
    pain and, 149, 150, 175
    prevention, 6
    recurrence of, 178
    resources, 107-117
    risky behaviors due to, 89
    smoking and, 125-126
    specialized care, 13, 59-69
    staging, 27-29
    stress and, 89
    support groups for, 77, 92, 128, 149
    survivor, 74, 169
    survivorship, 8
    symptoms of, 29-31
    treatment for, 21-27, 98-106
    types of, 19
cancer-free, 3, 9
cancerous cells, 7, 23-25, 179
cancerous mass, 23
cancer-related fatigue (CRF), 148
carbon monoxide, 126
carcinogens, 20, 34, 125, 157
carcinoma, 19, 28
    transitional cell, 19
caregiver burnout, 65, 144
caregiver support, 60, 63
caregivers, 59, 62, 128
    and family members, 202-204
    challenges facing, 62
    primary, 65
category, 80
    chronic, 135
    health, 78, 142
cell:
    abnormal, 17, 29, 157
    abnormality, 28
    balance, 17
    death, 7, 24
    division, 17, 20
    growth, 15, 24
    healthy, 17, 19, 24-25, 125, 148
    leftover, 179
    mother, 18
    mutation of, 20
    proliferation, 25
    replenishments of, 17
cervical cancer, 8
checkpoint inhibitors, 24
checkpoints, 17
checkups, 6, 31
chemo drugs, 136
chemotherapy, 24, 101-102
    drugs, 134
    dry mouth and, 177
    hair loss and, 176

late effects of, 173-175
pain and, 149, 150
palliative, 62, 63
second cancers and, 180
side effects of, 143-151
traditional, 25, 134
vitamin C and, 53
child, 96, 203
childcare, 41
childhood, 114
children, 19, 55, 66, 112, 145, 195
burden on, 109, 194
communication with, 198
inability to have, 177
raising, 151
young, 202
chills, 180
chiropractic care, 55, 56
chronic disease, or illness, 11, 109
cancer as a, 135-137
chronic inflammation, 157
chronic stress, 89
cigarettes, 6, 126
cisplatin, 174
clergy, 64, 65, 199, 202
clinical trials, 36-45
admission to, 37, 41-42
cost of, 42
definition of, 37, 38
phases of, 38-40
risks and benefits of, 42
safety in, 41-45
stress involved in, 42
coaching, 159-160
group, 151
see also cancer coaching
codeine, 151
cognitive rehabilitation, 173
collaboration, 112, 162
colon cancer, 19
colonoscopy, 7
comfort care, 60, 201
see also palliative care
communication, 55, 66, 100, 160
avoid, 203
channels of, 197
establishing, 105

focused, 55
importance of, 162, 193, 197-199
lack of, 57
with family, 198
with your doctor, 57
with your partner, 197-198
community, 68, 114, 156, 163
medical, 18, 34, 60, 99, 177
religious, 108, 114, 116
resources, 108
services, 77
support, 75
compassionate drug use, 43-45
compassionate presence, 114
complementary and alternative medicine, 46-58
complementary therapy, 47-50
benefits of, 47
effectiveness of, 57, 99
insurance and, 54, 56
safety and, 53
who pays for, 54
complete remission, 32, 133, 142
complications, 4, 44, 136
digestive, 89
emotional trauma, 4
lung, 178
medication, 136
overweight, 124
physical challenges, 147
comprehensive cancer centers, 111
confusion, 60, 87, 100
feelings of, 146 -147
final days and, 193-196
negative feelings and, 147
second opinion and, 105
constipation, 150, 173
continuum, 3-14, 91, 119
best position on the, 169
cancer, 4, 182
cancer-care, 112
definition, 5
health across the, 5-9
stages of the, 6-9, 90
starting point of the, 80
your position on the, 9-10, 73,

80
control, 6, 11, 34, 92, 113
    lymphedema, 122
    nausea, 48
    pain, 151
    side effects, 38
    symptom, 55, 66
    weight, 68, 124-125, 174
conventional medicine, 46, 54, 57
cooperative groups, 38, 111
coping, 122, 128, 196
    in the extended phase, 137-139
    in the permanent phase, 169, 180
    strategies, 89, 126, 185
    with psychological stress, 90
counseling, 42, 90, 119, 137, 151
    emotional, 13
    for emotional distress, 90, 121
    professional, 78, 120-122, 173
    psychological, 196
    spiritual, 69, 115
coverage, 42, 54-56
    insurance, 66, 101,190
cultural backgrounds, 133
curative treatment, 104
    vs., palliative 60-63
cytokines, 119
cytostatic, 25
cytotoxic, 25

D

"do not resuscitate" (DNR) order, 201
dance, 52
death, 3, 8, 65, 74
    accept, 200
    after, 14
    before, 59, 79
    cell, 17, 20, 23-24,
    early, 89
    emotions and, 193-204
    fear of, 195
    feeling alone and, 195
    of a child, 19
    time of, 197

    see also end of life
debulking, 22
decisions, 8, 47, 75, 90, 100
    CAM, 57
    end of life, 115
    health, 10
    legal, 200
    treatment, 12, 99, 103
deep breathing, 49, 93, 145
defective cells, 6
denial (emotions), 91, 120, 145
dentist, 177
depression, 62, 119
    anxiety and, 195
    diagnosis and, 143-144
    during the final days, 193-194
    exercise and, 123-124
    fear and, 120
    isolating yourself and, 116
    massage therapy and, 48-49
    medications for, 90
    music therapy and, 49
    negative thinking and, 92
    neglected, 144
    recognizing, 91-92
    reduced levels of, 89-90
    sorrow and, 145
    stress and, 126
    yoga and, 49
detachment, 115
determination, 3, 43, 191
developmental state, 15
diabetes, 126, 135
diagnosis report, 93-96
    anatomy of the, 94-95
diagnosis:
    after, 68-69, 86
    and treatment, 185-191
    blame and, 88, 92
    burden because of, 4
    CAM and, 55
    confusion and, 146
    emotional shock and, 87-90, 163
    emotional support after, 92
    expected challenges and, 99-101

get more info about your, 96, 97
impact of, 15
manage the shock of, 90-93
palliative care and, 59-63
physical reaction to, 86, 92
questions about, 31-34, 88
report, 93-96
resources and, 112-117
staging during, 28
survivorship and, 8-9
understand your, 14, 17, 89-97
diagnostic surgery, 21-22
diarrhea, 25, 27, 150
diet, 13, 54, 122
- balance your, 124
- balanced, 123, 156, 174, 178
- follow-up plan and, 140
- healthy, 173, 178
- *see also* nutrition
dietary ACTs, 52
dietary supplements, *see* supplements
dietary, 46, 52, 55
dietician, *see* nutritionist
digestive complications, 89
digestive system, 19
discover resources, 75, 108-117
distant recurrence, 179
distress, 89, 90, 112-115
DNA, 18-23
doctors:
- addiction concerns and, 151
- alternative therapies and, 13, 46
- biased, 58
- choosing, 112
- clinical trials and, 36-45
- communicating with, 94, 96
- expertise of, 100
- follow-up visits to, 190
- pain control and, 138, 150-151
- questions to ask, 33
- recommendations for, 97
- second opinion and, 105
dosage, 174
dose, 25, 37, 174, 176
- safe, 39
dreams, 138, 152, 201-202
loss of, 195
drugmaker, 44
drugs:
- antiseizure, 151
- chemotherapy, 24, 46, 133-136, 174-175
- classes of, 150-151
- compassionate use, 43-44
- investigational, 37, 41, 43-44
- potent, 24
- testing of, 39
- unapproved, 44
dry mouth, 48, 176, 177
durable power of attorney, 201
durable remission, 32
dying, 193-204

E

early screening, 3-5, 7, 9, 12, 163
eating, *see also* diet
education, 7, 15, 79, 140, 156
- patient, 57
electrons, 23
eligibility criteria, 40, 42
eliminating a body part, 171
eliminating disputes, 200
eliminating obstacles, 7
eliminating symptoms, 62
emotional, 15, 33, 60, 68
- burden, 65
- challenges, 91, 127
- changes, 112, 120, 173
- counseling, 13, 69
- healing, 147
- needs, 61, 64
- numbness, 120, 146
- outburst, 194
- paralysis, 86
- reactions, 86, 158
- recovery, 115
- scars, 99
- shock, 87-90, 93
- state, 42, 76, 79
- stress, 13, 158
- support, 91, 92, 138
- trauma, 4, 75, 76, 92, 112

emotions, *see* feelings
employment, 61, 109, 147
empowering, 161
end of life, 60-63, 79, 192-204
endoscope, 22
enemas, 52
energy, 148-149, 158, 186
    body's, 31
    therapies, 52
environmental factors, 20, 34, 157
enzymes, 25, 52
epithelial, 19
erectile dysfunction, 177
esophagus, 19, 22
ethical obligations, 57
evaluate your life, 181-191
excisional, *see* biopsy
exclusion criteria, 42
exercise, 123-128
    amount recommendations, 123-124
    benefits of, 122-124
    bone problems and, 175
    fatigue and, 148
    follow-up plan and, 140, 156
    gentle movement, 49
    heart problems and, 174
    lymphedema and, 122, 172
    stress and, 90, 126-127
    tai chi, 49
    yoga, 55, 157
expanded patient access, 43
expanded scar formation, 172
experimental treatments, 37
    see also clinical trials
extended phase, 73, 76, 131-140
    balance your diet in the, 124
    categorize your health in the, 131-140
    control your weight in the, 124-124
    exercise in the, 123-124
    reduce stress in the, 126-127
    rest well in the, 125
    stop drinking alcohol in the, 126
    transitioning to, 127
extended survival, 4
extended survivorship phase, *see* extended phase
external radiation, 23
eye problems, 175
eyes, 30, 175, 196
    dehydrated, 175

F

faith, 114-116, 199, 202
families, 62, 143, 202
family history, 23, 31, 140, 172
fatigue, 148-149
    after treatment and, 143, 157
    and exercise, 123
    appetite and, 173
    chemotherapy and, 174
    immunotherapy and, 25
    pain and, 147
    radiation therapy and, 150, 176
    surgery and, 150
fatty acids, 124
FDA, 37-44, 53, 58
fear, 120, 142, 169, 151, 188
    manage the, 189
    of addiction, 151
    of recurrence, 78, 142, 144
    of the unknown and death, 146, 193-195
feelings, 88-91, 142
    accepting your, 91
    analyze the, 185
    as an obstacle, 89
    helpless, 89
    identify your, 90
    negative thoughts and, 142-143
    of being alone, 193
    of confusion, 146-147
    of isolation, 161
    of loneliness, 115, 185
    of sorrow, 120, 145-146
    of uncertainty, 189
    of worry, 144-145
    positive thoughts and, 142
fertility, 89, 173, 177
    see also infertility

fever, 25, 31, 178
final days, 192-194
financial help, 42, 93, 116
financial issues, 4
fish oil, 55
five-year survival rate, 4, 31
fluid, 148, 173, 201
Fox Chase Cancer Center, 114
free of cancer, 32
friends, 62, 88, 108, 149
    communication with, 197-198
    help from, 11, 93
    mixed reactions and, 184
    support of, 114, 117
funeral directors, 65
follow-up, 122, 140, 163
    appointment, 127, 146
    care plan, 128, 139, 143, 179
    visits, 76, 189-190
food, 173, 178, 194, 196
fruits, 52, 124, 174
farewell, 201-204
final days, 192
    communications during the, 198-199
    emotions during the, 193-195
fear, 120, 151, 188
Food and Drug Administration, 12, 43

G

gallbladder, 150
gamma rays, 23
gastrointestinal, 25
gender, 34, 42, 121
genes, 20, 25, 95
    onco, 32
    suppressor, 32
genetic mutations, 32
genetic, 6, 27, 32, 35, 172
Gerson regimen, 52
ginger, 48
ginseng, 53
goals, 37, 77, 124, 152
    deciding on, 104-105
    treatment, 62

grade, 33, 94-95
graft-versus-tumor, 27
green tea, 53
grief, 194-195
grieving, 145, 203
grocery store, 53, 149-150
gross description, 94
group, 44, 46, 76, 137
    advocacy, 161
    coaching, 151
    members, 149
    settings, 49, 90
    support, 15
growth, 23, 134, 172
    abnormal, 18
    cancer, 25-27
    cell, 16, 24
guidance, 10, 86, 147
guided imagery, 48
guilt, 145, 193-194

H

hair cells, 176
hair loss, 121, 174, 176
hallucination, 196-197
head and neck cancer, 48
head, radiation to the, 177
health care providers, 55, 108-109
health care resources, *see* resources
health insurance, 44, 56, 160
health promotions, 5, 77
hearing loss, 174
heart disease, 126, 135
heart problems, 121, 147, 174
heart, 116
herbal medicines, 53
herbs, 13, 48, 52
high blood pressure, 25-26
high doses, 23, 26-27, 176-177
    of supplements, 53
HMO's, 68
Hodgkin's lymphoma, 19
home health, 64, 66
homeopathy, 51
honesty, 197, 204
hormone receptors, 95

hormone therapy, 26, 102, 134
hormones, 26, 88, 133
hospice care, 63-68
    time limitations for, 64
hospitals, 66, 123, 187
    pastoral services in, 116
HPV, 205
humorous, 91
hypnosis, 48, 151
hypnotherapy, 47

I

ibuprofen, 150
identical twin, 26
image, 49
imaging, 190
immune cells, 119
immune system, 19, 24, 157
    activate the, 119
    damage to the, 29
    healthy, 34
    progression and the,
    suppressed, 158
    weakened, 20, 89
    see also immune cells
immunity, 34, 54
immunotherapy, 24-25
    see also immune system
impairment, 4, 9, 62, 119, 200
in situ, 29
incisional biopsy, 21
inclusion criteria, 42
incurable cancer, 138
infection, 19, 25, 34, 102, 169
infertility, *see* fertility
inflammation, 119, 158
informed decisions, 8, 12, 100
inpatient facility, 65
insurance, 41-44, 56, 93, 190
    see also coverage
integrative medicine, 54, 58
intensive treatment, 113
intensive, 92
interaction, 116, 126, 162
interdisciplinary, 64
Internet, 96, 162

intervention, 50, 90, 119, 113
intestinal tract, 22
intimacy, 173, 198
intravenously, 24
intravesical, 24
invasive surgery, 23
invasive, 96
investigation drugs, 37, 41, 41-45
investigational treatment, 41
irradiated area, 23

J

jaundice, 30
job and family, 42
Joint Commission, 111
joint pain, 175
joint problems, 175
juice, 52

K

keyhole, 23
kidney, 150, 174, 201

L

laboratory, 94, 111
laetrile, 53
lasers, 172
laughter, 203
legal obligations, 57
legal, 61
    advance directives, 200
lens, 95
    eye, 175
lesion, 18
leukemia, 19, 27, 134, 135
leukocytes, 27
life's meaning, 182, 195
lifestyle, 54, 123, 137, 142
    adjustments, 79, 92
    changes, 4, 10, 147
    habits, 6, 15-21, 122
    healthy, 89, 124
light:

exercises, 123
sensitivity to, 175
walk, 149
workout, 49, 172
liver enzymes, 25
liver, 25, 179
living will, 201
localized cancers, 22
localized, 23, 29, 97
long-term, 27, 33, 123
    care facility, 60, 66
    chronic stress, 89
    disabilities, 147
    memory loss, 173
    side effects, 9, 27, 40
    survival, 7
lung cancer, 6, 53
lung problems, 177
    smoking and, 178
lung, 18, 124, 179
lymph fluid, 175
lymph nodes, 22, 28, 95, 179
    regional, 29
lymphatic system, 18-19
lymphedema, 172
lymphocytes, 19
lymphoma, 19
    primary CNS, 20

M

magnetic resonance imaging (MRI), 133
maintained remission, 76, 132, 134 135
malignancy, 18, 169
mammogram, 7
massage therapy, 48-49, 52, 93
massage, 123, 151, 170
mastectomy, 22, 23, 121, 150
Mayo Clinic, 125, 177
meats, 124
Medicaid, 68
medical community, 18, 34, 60, 177
medical insurance, 190
medical, 4, 68
    director, 64, 66

facility, 63
information, 60
institutions, 75, 100
practice, 47, 51
professionals, 12
team, 67
terminology, 86, 93, 162
tests, 39, 41
treatment, 50
Medicare Hospice Advantage, 64
Medicare Hospice Benefit, 64
Medicare, 64, 66, 68, 190
medications, 34, 49, 93, 119, 125
    addiction to, 151
    anxiety and, 195
    fatigue and, 148, 157
    for depression, 90
    memory loss and, 173
    off-the-shelve, 87
    pain, 23, 138, 151
    stress and, 126
    strong pain, 150-151
melanoma, 7, 31
melatonin, 53
memory loss, 173
menopause, 27, 175, 177
mental health, 15, 91
mental imagery, 93
mental interventions, 144
metastasis, 175, 206
    distant, 79
microscope, 94, 180
microscopic description, 95
mind-body, 52
    practices, 157-159
mineral supplements, 53
minimally invasive surgery, 23
mitotic rate, 94, 95
mole, 7
molecular, 25, 32
monoclonal antibodies, 24
mood changes, 26
mood fluctuations, 122
mood, 61, 123
morbidity, 144
morphine, 151
motivation, 149, 160

mourning, 65
mouth, 23, 53, 126
    dry, 48, 176, 177
    sores, 27, 150, 174
    ulcers, 18
moving forward, 189-191
MRI scans, 133
multidisciplinary, 4, 13, 60, 162
multidisease, 2, 15
multivitamin, 124
muscle relaxation, 50, 93
muscle weakness, 174
muscles, 21, 31, 49
mushroom extract, 53
music, 52, 149
    listening to, 173
    relaxing, 156, 197
    therapy, 49
mutations, 20, 32
myeloma and multiple myeloma, 19, 27

N

median duration, 62
National Cancer Institute, 7, 38, 96, 113
National Clinical Trials Network, 111
National Coalition for Cancer Survivorship, 96, 161
National Institute of Health, 133
National Institute of Mental Health, 91
natural defenses, 17
natural products, 46-47, 52-56
naturopathy, 51
nausea, 25-27, 48, 51, 119, 150
neck cancer, 48
needles, 48
negative emotions, 160
    and depression, 117
    severity of, 90
negative thoughts, 120, 142
neoadjuvant therapy, 26
neoplasm, 18
nerve damage, 136, 147, 171, 177

nerve injury, 150
nerve pain, 150
nerve, 22
nervous system, 19
neurological, 158
neuropathy, 150
nutrition, 139, 201
    fatigue and, 148
nipple, 30, 150
nocebo, 50
noncurative, 13, 59, 68-69
non-Hodgkin's lymphoma, 19
nonpatients, 12, 124, 146
numbness, 120, 146
nurses, 60-66
nursing homes, 65-68
nurture, 156-163
nutrient, 17, 124, 178
nutritional plan, 93, 125, 145
nutritionist, 93, 124-125, 148, 173
nuts, 124, 173

O

obesity, 7, 34
obvious description, 94
occupational therapist, 148
old age, 152
older generation, 151
older patients, 151, 172
oncogenes, 32
oncologists, 12, 62, 110
oncology certified nurses, 97, 139
oncology nutritionist, 124
oncology physical therapist, 57, 175
oncology, 39, 52
oophorectomy, 23
ophthalmologist, 175
opioids, 150
orally, 24
organs, 19, 30, 121
orgasm, 177
osteopathic manipulation, 52, 55
osteopathic medicine, 13
osteoporosis, 175
outpatient clinic, 60
outpatient treatments, 112

outpatient, 112
ovarian cancer, 23, 135
overeating, 89
oxycodone, 151
oxygen therapy, 178

P

pain: 138
    abdominal and back, 30
    acute, 150
    causes of physical, 149
    chemotherapy and, 24
    chest, 174
    chronic, 147, 150, 157, 173
    exercise and, 123
    fatigue and, 148, 157
    hypnotherapy and, 48
    medications for, 23, 150, 201
    no improvement in handling, 158
    palliative surgery and, 22
    prevention surgery and, 23
    radiation therapy and, 23
    specialist, 151
palliative care, 60-63
palliative chemotherapy, 62-63
pancreatic tumors, 30, 31
pap smear, 7
partial remission, 133
participation, 108
    in your health, 10, 110
    patient, 11
partner, 121, 197
pastor, *see* clergy
pathologists, 22, 94
pathology report, 22, 28, 86, 93
patient education, 57
patient:
    advocate, 156, 162
    care, 47, 65
    dreams, 104, 138, 195, 201
    involvement, 10
    participation and confidence, 11
    treatment plan, 44
patients, cancer, 33, 65, 104, 146

challenges facing, 147
diet and, 124
fatigue and, 49
hair loss in, 176
life purpose and, 182
newly diagnosed, 170
physical activity for, 123
social support for, 116
terminal, 62
pelvic area, 177
permanent phase, 8, 78, 167
personality issues, 174
personality, 120, 143
personalized medicine, 27
pharmaceutical. 134
pharmacist, 60, 65
photodynamic therapy, 102
physical state, 121
physical trauma, 79
physician, 43, 60, 99, 110
pituitary gland, 177
placebo and placebo effect, 50, 51
plasma cells, 19
platelets, 27
positive attitude, 128, 156
positive relationship, 109
positive thinking, 87
potent opioids, 151
pranayama, 157, 158
prevention, 6
primary cancer, 22, 73, 178
primary care, 10, 91, 140
priorities, 55, 184, 186
prognosis, 33
progression, 32
prostate cancer, 26, 135, 190
prostate, 11, 26
prostatectomy, 121
prostate-specific antigen (PSA), 190
protein, 124, 173, 178
protocol, 17, 40
PSA (prostate-specific antigen), 190
psychological state, 119
psychologists, 88, 113
psychosocial support, 15
psychosocial, 4, 11, 144, 168

Q

quality of life, 37, 60-67, 157

R

radiation, or radiation therapy:
    and pain, 149
    direct, 178
    dosage, 140
    expected challenges and, 99
    extra beam, 102
    heart problems and, 174
    in or near the tumor, 2
    in women, 177
    late effects of, 176-178
    risk of occurrence and, 133
    safety issues and, 53
    second cancers and, 180
    session, 23
radioactive, 23
radiotherapy, 24, 48
recurrence, 178-180
red blood cells, 27
reflection, 55, 157
regression, 32
rehabilitation, 9, 111, 147
    cognitive, 173
relaxation techniques, 50, 90, 93
relief, 91, 169
    financial, 37
    dry mouth, 177
    symptom, 104
religion, 49, 113-116, 199
remission, 32
    cancer-free vs., 133
    complete, 32, 133, 142
    durable remission, 32
    maintained, 134-135
    partial, 133, 135
    spontaneous, 32
    treatment-free, 132-133
    types of, 133, 134
risk factors, 31, 34, 97
    exposure to, 9
    learn about, 14

reproductive organs, 177
resistance strength training, 175
resources, 227-244
    psychological, 112
    spiritual, 113
    social, 116
respite care, 65
response rate, 39, 62
responsibility, 7, 43, 57
rest, 125, 149,
restate your priorities, 192-204

S

sadness, 138
safe dosage, 39
safe sex, 6
sampling variations, 95
sampling, 95
sarcoma, 19, 150
scalpels, 21
scarring, 23, 172
    and age, 172
school, 163, 203
    children, 112
second cancer, 78, 168, 179
second opinion, 43, 57,
    advantages, 8
    conflict in, 105
second primary cancer, 126
self-care, 12, 56, 156
self-repair, 157
sex and intimacy, 198
sex, 143
sexual functions, 121, 173
shark cartilage, 52, 53
siblings, 204
single patient access, 43
signals, 193, 196
skin cancer, 7, 18, 24
skin changes, 121
skin rashes, 174
skin, 16-25, 48, 121, 173, 196
sleep disturbances, 157
sleep during end of life, 196
sleep, 89, 125
smoking, 20, 89

follow-up plan and, 140
lung problems and, 178
quitting of, 68
stop, 125-126
social interactions, 116
social worker, 90, 113
socioeconomic state, 7, 15
sorrow, 195
    feelings of, 120, 145-146
soul, 157
sound, 49
specialized cancer care, 60-69
specialized tests, 131
speech therapist, 174
sperm, 177
spinal cord, 19, 22, 28
spinal fluid, 24
spiritual counseling, 69, 115
spiritual distress, 120, 146
spirituality, 49, 113-116
spontaneous remission, 32
stable health, 6
stage of cancer, 95, 140, 148
staging surgery, 22
staging, 8, 17, 101
    cancer, 26
    diagnosis and, 89, 94
    TNM, 28, 29
standard therapy, 24, 41, 57
stem cell transplants, 26, 27
steroids, 151, 172, 178
stimulations, 48, 157
stomach, 22, 173, 195
stool, 180
stress hormones, 88
stress, 88-89
stressors, 93, 143, 146
stroke, 126
suicide, 17, 144
sun, 6, 20,
sunlight, 176
supplements, 52, 53
support groups, 77, 92, 122, 126, 149
support systems, 9, 92, 128, 189
supportive care, 60, 137
    see also palliative care
suppressor genes, 32

surgery:
    diagnostic, 21
    late term effects of, 171-173
    palliative and curative, 22
    prevention, 23
    reconstructive, 122, 172
    side-effects of, 12
    staging, 22
surveillance, 79, 140
survival rate, 4, 31, 103
    statistic and, 103
survival, 27, 63, 89, 105, 126, 144
    chances of, 27, 31, 105
    five-year, 31
    improving the, 39
    prolong, 61
survivor, 8, 74, 140, 191
survivorship care plan, 139, 140
survivorship planning, 9
symptom management, 60
    see also palliative care
symptoms of cancer, 29-31
syndrome, 175
synoptic summary, 95
systemic, 24

T

tai chi, 49-50
tension, 198
terminology, 62
    medical, 86, 93, 100, 162
    war, 3
testicles, 177
testosterone, 177
throat, 19, 126
thymus extract, 53
thyroid, 27, 176
tissue damage, 149
tissue mass, 18
tissue, 22, 29, 94
TNM staging system, 28, 29
tobacco, 7
toxic, 25
toxicity, 39, 48
traditional Chinese medicine therapy, 48

transitional cell carcinoma, 19
transitional phase, 76
transitional phase, *see* extended phase
transplants, 27
    bone marrow, 148
    stem cell, 26
trauma, 92, 112
treatment options, 21-27
    deciding on goals, 104
    decision time, 102
    expected challenges, 99
    navigate your, 98
    second opinion, 105
treatments decisions, 12
treatments:
    advances in, 33
    bio-electromagnetic based, 52
    choices, 21, 60, 90, 101
    common, 9
    conventional, 46
    curative, 104
    decide on the, 97
    decisions, 12
    diagnosis and, 15, 95, 113
    experimental, 37
    goals of, 62
    hair loss and cancer, 121
    halting, 137
    hospice care, 64
    investigational drugs and, 41
    investigational, 41
    mind-body, 158
    mix of, 15, 18, 21, 76
    most common cancer, 9
    new, 41
    prognosis and, 33
    proper, 54
    safety issues and, 53
    spiritual practices and, 116
    value in choosing, 159
trust, 64, 103, 116
tumor margin, 94,
tumor markers, 95
tumor markers, 95
tumors, 31
    benign and malignant, 18
    brain, 7, 28

Tylenol, 150

U

ulcers, 150
    mouth, 18
uncertainty, 138, 146, 189
unconventional treatments, 47, 151
unfinished business, 199-202
    accomplish unfinished tasks, 201
    advance directives, 200-201
    assess your life, 202
    go back to religion, 202
urinary problems, 89, 175
urine, 180
uterus, 19, 22

V

vaccination, 205
vaccines, 24
vaginal dryness, 26
vegetables, 53, 124. 174
vegetarian, 52
vein, 24, 31
viruses, 20, 34
vitamin B-17, 53
vitamin C, 53
vitamins, 46, 52-55, 124, 148
volunteering, 156, 159-161

W

warning signals of dying, 196
wart, 30
weak bones. 22
weak medications, 150
weight, 124-125
western world, 52
white blood cells, 19, 24, 27
whole grains, 124, 174
wigs, 188
will, *see* living will
World Health Organization, 6, 7
worry, 120, 144-145, 163, 195

financial, 61
see also anxiety

X
xerostomia, 177
X-rays, 23, 28

Y
yoga, 49, 157
yogic breathing strategies, 157
younger generation, 198

www.ingramcontent.com/pod-product-compliance
Lightning Source LLC
Chambersburg PA
CBHW070914030426
42336CB00014BA/2414